Reviews

"Sharon Masinelli, P[...] x questions
about heart disease [...] for lay people.
Her advice is reasona[...] uring. I highly recommend this book to eve[...] as heart disease as well as to
their families."

Doreen C. Parkhurst, MD, FACEP

"Ms. Masinelli's book is right on. Her concise explanation of
heart disease and its treatment should prove very beneficial to
patients from every background. I will certainly recommend it
for my practice. Great job, Sharon."

Mark Moronell, MD, FACC

"Sharon Masinelli PA-C has written a book all patients with coronary heart disease & their families should read. She has taken a
very difficult subject & condensed it into a very readable text for
the average person. The information & advice she gives is accurate, timely & truly reflects the current standard."

Richard B Fien, MD, MPH, FACC

What to Do When You Have Heart Disease

What to Do When You Have Heart Disease

A Handy Guide for Living Well with Heart Disease

Sharon Masinelli, MCMS, PA-C

iUniverse, Inc.
New York   Bloomington

What to Do When You Have Heart Disease
A Handy Guide for Living Well with Heart Disease

iUniverse books may be ordered through booksellers or by contacting:

iUniverse
1663 Liberty Drive
Bloomington, IN 47403
www.iuniverse.com
1-800-Authors (1-800-288-4677)

ISBN: 978-1-4401-8473-4 (pbk)
ISBN: 978-1-4401-8472-7 (ebk)
ISBN: 978-1-4401-8471-0 (hbk)

Library of Congress Control Number: 2009911483

Printed in the United States of America

iUniverse rev. date: 12/7/2009

Credits: Special thanks to Edward Sicotte for the illustrations, Joyce Pagan for her editing expertise, my husband for his love and support, and most especially the cardiologists and office staff who trained me and provided the knowledge base for this book.

Portions of this book were derived from my article "How do I control my heart failure?" published in the March 2009 issue of the Journal of the American Academy of Physician Assistants. Express written permission was obtained prior to publication.

This book is dedicated to my wonderful family and especially to my caring husband, Bob. Thank you to all who encouraged me throughout the writing process. Most of all, thank you, God, for giving me the strength, knowledge, and endurance to complete this book!

In loving memory of my sweet mother, Carol, who passed away before this book could be published.

Contents

Introduction:
Finding the Information You Need

If you are reading this book, you most likely want to know more about heart disease. In the fast pace of today's hospitals and doctors' offices, most people who receive a diagnosis of heart disease are left with many questions about heart disease and its treatment. This book is designed to help you when you are wondering what to do next.

You can certainly read this book from cover to cover and learn as much as you can about heart disease. However, in case you prefer to go directly to the information you need at any given moment, here is a quick guide for where you can find commonly needed information.

- Do you want to know more about stents and bypass surgery?
  - o Chapter 6 discusses the procedures and recovery times.

- Are you still in the hospital or have you been released within the past few days?
    - Chapters 7 and 8 deal with immediate after-hospital care.

- Have you had heart disease for a while and want to avoid another trip to the hospital?
    - Chapter 9 is a great place to start; then read through the chapter titles and review the tables at the back of the book.

- Do you need to learn more about the medicines you are taking?
    - Chapter 10 gives specific information about the medicines used to treat heart disease. There is also a medicine list at the end of this book that lists the generic and brand names of the drugs.

- Do you need to know more about cholesterol?
    - Chapter 12 talks about what you need to know as a person with heart disease.

- Are you concerned about recognizing the signs of another heart problem?
  - Chapter 15 spells out the signs and symptoms to be concerned about. Another helpful tool is the table included at the back of the book, "What to Do When You Have Chest Pain."

- Do you have heart failure and need to know more about how to control it?
  - Chapter 16 will teach you the basics of living well with heart failure.

- Are you looking for information on a heart-healthy diet?
  - Chapter 18 gets you started in the right direction.

- Are you looking for tips on finding less-expensive medicine?
  - Chapter 22 is just what you need.

- Do you want to look for a specific subject or term to learn more about it?

- Look in the index to find the pages with the information you need.

- Do you just want to find basic information quickly?
  - The tables at the back of the book sum up the basic information provided by this book, or you can read through the chapter titles for the subjects that interest you.

Chapter 1
Seventy Million Americans

The moment when a person first finds out that they have heart disease can be a hazy one. Some people discover that they have heart disease during a visit with the doctor. Others have the misfortune of lying in a hospital bed when the diagnosis is made. Either way, life may never be the same again. Many cannot fully realize the extent of what is happening because it is an unexpected event.

Chances are that you or a loved one has heart disease. Heart disease is very common and affects as many as seventy million Americans. The American Heart Association estimated that 770,000 people had a heart attack in 2008. Just looking at the numbers, one can easily say that heart disease is an epidemic. Large organizations have taken on the task of trying to improve the statistics. Advances in modern medicine and public education about treating the risk factors have resulted in a decline in the risk of death. However, heart disease is still the number one cause of death in the United States.

Most people know that heart disease is a very serious and life-threatening problem. Many important questions have to be answered after you learn that you have heart disease. Probably the first questions people think of are the following:

- What happens next?
- Am I going to die soon?
- What can I do to make my heart better?

Just when you think your situation is hopeless, the cardiologist arrives to tell you that something *can* be done. Coronary stents, bypass surgery, or medication can prevent significant heart damage and save lives. This book is intended to help people learn about heart disease and be able to get the best treatment possible.

What motivates me to write about this subject? First and foremost, I am a physician assistant (PA) who specialized in cardiology (the study and treatment of the heart). Most of my patients were referred to as hospital follow-ups. This means that the person was recently released from the hospital after having a new heart problem and is seeing me in the office for post-discharge care. I believe that spending time with these new patients and teaching them about heart disease and how to take better care of their heart is important.

On a more personal note, my grandfather died as a result of a heart attack when I was a child. In addition to that tragedy, my father also had a heart attack when I was in high school. I have personally lived through the agony and confusion that follows when heart disease strikes a loved one.

Chapter 2
What Is Heart Disease?

Heart disease can be defined in many ways. The American Heart Association defines cardiovascular disease as high blood pressure, a previous heart attack, angina, a previous stroke, heart failure, or a birth defect in the heart. Patients who have problems with heart valves or an irregular heart rhythm may also be considered to have heart disease. This book focuses primarily on people who have had a previous heart attack, angina, one or more blockages in the heart arteries, and heart failure.

The condition of blocked arteries of the heart is called coronary artery disease (CAD) or coronary heart disease (CHD). This means that a plaque formed in one or more of the arteries leading to the heart. Some imaging studies of the heart can calculate the percentage of blockage. A blockage is called a stenosis. Blood flow is impaired by plaque buildup, but the blockage is usually not considered to be significant until the plaque blocks 70 percent or more of the artery. The large main artery of the heart, called the left main artery, is considered to have a significant blockage when the plaque reaches 50 percent or more. A blockage of 100 percent is a completely blocked artery; no blood can get through at all. This is called a total occlusion. If a fully blocked artery is called chronically occluded, this means it has been blocked for a long time.

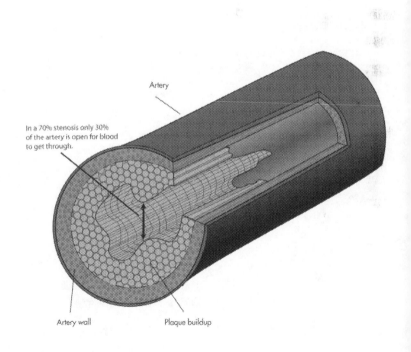

Artery

In a 70% stenosis only 30% of the artery is open for blood to get through.

Artery wall

Plaque buildup

70% Blockage

70 percent blockage

Sharon Masinelli, MCMS, PA-C

The exact process of how plaque forms in the arteries is still somewhat of a mystery. Many theories and studies have revealed much of the process; but surprisingly, the full extent of what occurs during the plaque formation is unknown. If we did know exactly how it happens, heart disease probably would not be the number one cause of death in the United States!

Even though we do not definitively know what causes heart disease, there are important risk factors that can increase the chance of developing heart disease. The following conditions can significantly increase a person's risk for heart disease:

- High blood pressure
- Diabetes
- High cholesterol
- Family history of heart attacks
- Smoking
- Increasing age

When a stenosis blocks 70 percent or more of the artery, the person may develop symptoms like chest pain and shortness of breath. Chest pain caused by a stenosis is called angina. This is usually only diagnosed in someone who has a known heart blockage. An angina attack is typically brought on when a person does heavy physical activity. The pain is felt when the heart has a greater need for blood, such as when walking up the stairs. Enough blood may be flowing past the blockage when you are at rest, but as soon as the heart is put under stress—or needs to pump blood faster—you feel pain because the blood supply to the heart muscle is decreased. Stable angina means that the pain goes away with rest. Unstable angina means that the pain gets worse, lasts longer, and is not relieved by rest.

A complete blockage may be caused by a clot and result in a heart attack. A heart attack is also called a myocardial infarction (MI). During a heart attack, inflammation and the body's response to injury play key roles. It is believed that the process starts with development of a crack in the plaque. The body responds to the crack the same way it would for a cut on the skin. Platelets are sent to the artery to form a clot or scab. Unfortunately, areas with plaque do not have enough space for the clot. Instead, the clot becomes a plug in the artery, and blood can no longer get through the artery at all. If the blood flow is stopped for too long, the heart tissue begins to die.

Sharon Masinelli, MCMS, PA-C

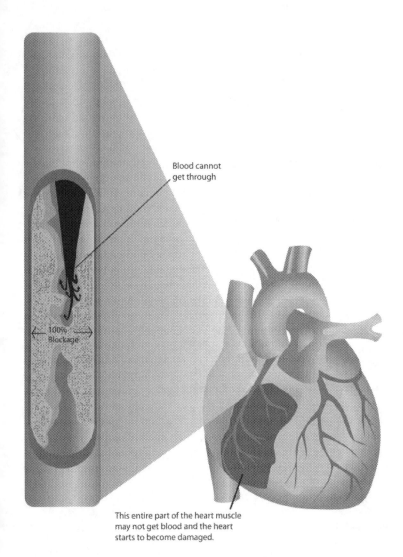

Blood cannot
get through

100%
Blockage

This entire part of the heart muscle
may not get blood and the heart
starts to become damaged.

Complete blockage during MI

In addition to blockages in the arteries, many heart
disease patients may progress to heart failure (also called

congestive heart failure, CHF, or HF). Heart failure occurs when the heart is weak and cannot pump out enough blood to the body. Sometimes heart failure can also be caused by the heart being unable to relax properly between beats. If the heart cannot relax, it cannot fill with enough blood to pump out to the body. Either way, the blood does not flow as well as it should and backs up into the lungs and the extremities. People with heart failure often have shortness of breath and swelling in the legs. Heart failure is discussed further in chapter 16.

Chapter 3
How Is Heart Disease Diagnosed?

Several tests are used to diagnose problems with the heart. Most commonly, people will undergo electrocardiography, or EKG, in the doctor's office. An EKG records the electrical impulses of the heart. This test has been done for more than a hundred years and is still the first step in evaluating anyone with chest pain. An EKG is performed by placing ten stickers or leads on the chest, arms, and legs. Generally, the EKG prints the results in less than a minute, so this is a quick and painless test; and an EKG gives plenty of information. It can identify such problems as irregular heart rhythms, previous or current heart attacks, and possible heart artery blockages. Unfortunately, an EKG alone cannot make a positive diagnosis of heart disease; additional tests are required to support the findings.

If someone has had an abnormal EKG result in the doctor's office, the next step is usually a stress test. The different types of stress tests are exercise EKG treadmill, exercise nuclear stress, chemical nuclear stress, and stress echocardiography. The type of stress test conducted will depend on how active the patient is. If the patient can walk well on a treadmill, an exercise EKG or exercise nuclear stress is usually conducted.

An exercise EKG treadmill test involves the patient walking or jogging on a treadmill while hooked up to an EKG machine. A plain exercise EKG uses only the information derived from the EKG to determine if something is wrong with the heart. This test is used to screen for heart disease; however, sometimes the results may be unreliable.

In order to obtain more information during an exercise EKG treadmill test, a nuclear scan may be ordered in conjunction with the treadmill test. This constitutes an exercise nuclear stress test. Small amounts of a nuclear isotope are injected through an IV (into a vein) and a scan or image of the heart is obtained before and after the exercise portion of the test. The nuclear isotope is absorbed by the heart muscle and can make the heart appear on a computer screen brightly lit up. The nuclear substance only "lights up" the parts of the heart muscle that are receiving blood through the arteries. If a portion of the heart does not light up on the scan, your doctor can assume that the artery leading to that part of the heart muscle has a blockage.

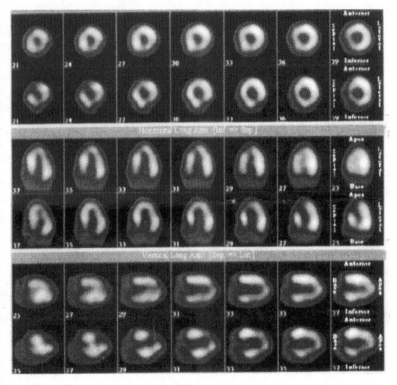

Nuclear image

If a patient is not able to walk independently on the treadmill, a chemical stress test is done. The chemical is a special drug administered through the IV that induces stress on the heart. Persantine, Lexiscan, adenosine, or dobutamine are the drugs that may be used. The side effects of these drugs are unpleasant but usually only last for a few minutes. The nuclear portion of the test is the same, including the nuclear isotope injection and obtaining the scan. Patients who cannot or do not want a nuclear stress test have the option of stress echocardiography. This involves obtaining an ultrasound image of the heart before and after exercise. No nuclear substances are used, and the results are often available much faster.

How reliable are the stress tests? The nuclear studies and stress echocardiography are fairly reliable; 85 percent or more of test results are true positives. A true positive is a result that accurately shows heart disease. How reliable the result is often depends on the type of equipment used, the physician reading the test, the size of the patient, and how well the heart was stressed. If a patient has a large chest or belly, his or her other anatomy may interfere with the quality of the pictures. Also, if the heart was not stressed well enough through exercise or chemicals, the result is less likely to accurately show heart disease.

The only affirmative way to actually see heart disease and diagnose it is with angiography, also known as heart catheterization. Angiography is an invasive procedure performed in a sterile surgery room or in a catheterization laboratory (cath lab) in the hospital. The patient puts on a hospital gown and is given mild sedatives before being taken into the cath lab. An artery in the groin is punctured with a needle, allowing a very small catheter to be threaded into the artery and up to the heart. Once the catheter reaches the heart, a dye is squirted into the various arteries on the heart. A continuous radiograph (x-ray) allows doctors and staff to watch the entire procedure on a television screen, and the patient is often awake for the entire time. The radiographic images (angiograms) will show if the heart arteries are narrow or blocked. As mentioned before, a blockage is usually not considered to be significant until 70 percent or more of the artery is blocked (or greater than 50 percent in the left main artery). The possibility of needing a stent (a wire mesh placed against the artery walls) or bypass surgery to fix significantly blocked areas will likely be discussed after the angiography is complete, when the patient has time to recover and consider all the options. A procedure is performed immediately on rare occasions when the degree of heart disease is critical.

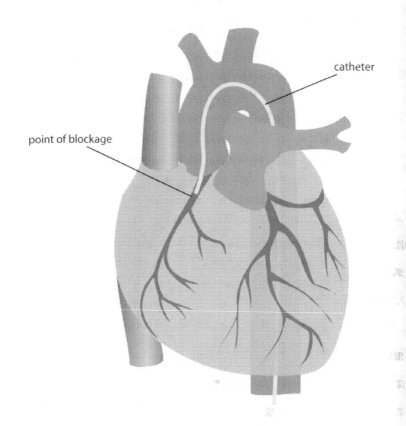

catheter

point of blockage

Cardiac catheterization

A noninvasive version of this test is called cardiac CT angiography. This test is not considered to be the "gold standard" for diagnosing heart disease, but improved techniques are making this a promising new technology. Cardiac CT angiography requires an IV and injection of a dye. The patient then undergoes a CT scan of the heart.

A radiologist or cardiologist interprets the angiograms after the test is completed; therefore, results may not be available for several days. CT angiography is currently less popular than other tests, probably because it is not covered by some health insurance plans. However, many patients hope the test will become one of the more widely used ways to identify heart disease in the future.

Your doctor can assume that you have heart disease or angina if you have typical symptoms; however, this cannot be confirmed without obtaining an angiogram. Many people believe they have angina without ever having undergone heart testing. The term may be inadvertently used to describe any suspicious chest pain. If you have ever been told that you have angina, you need to talk to your doctor about having the appropriate heart testing done. Chest pain caused by the heart should not be a guess! You need to know what is really going on so you can be treated properly.

In the emergency room (ER), a cardiologist may recommend skipping the stress test completely in favor of obtaining an angiogram. If the patient is having a heart attack or the symptoms of a significant blockage are enough of a concern, there is no point in wasting time. The patient is taken directly to the cath lab for angiography. Most likely, a stent is implanted within one to two hours.

Chapter 4
Standard of Care

Before discussing treatment options or cardiac workup, I must give a short disclaimer. For the most part, I am discussing medical decisions that are considered to be the standard of care. This means that the tests, medicines, and therapies are widely accepted by the medical community. Not only are these accepted, but this is the care that is expected to be given because these are proven to be of such great benefit. For example, aspirin has been shown to reduce the risk of a patient's having another heart attack by 25 percent. Large studies usually determine what should and should not be done for patients with heart disease. The standard is similar throughout the world, even in developing countries.

Treating patients to the highest standard of care is so important that national organizations have been formed just to develop and update the guidelines for care that are followed. For example, cardiologists and primary care physicians can volunteer to be evaluated by the National Committee for Quality Assurance

(NCQA). This group randomly reviews the charts of the doctor's heart disease and stroke patients to verify that the standard of care is being followed. If a majority of the doctor's patients meet the health standard goals, then the cardiologist or primary care physician is given a seal of approval from the NCQA.

With standard of care taken into consideration, I must also explain that each doctor is different and that each doctor's patient is different. Your doctor may think that you will not benefit from a particular test or treatment that is the standard of care. This does not mean that your doctor is giving you poor care. Treatment plans are customized for each patient. For example, the standard of care is to tell a person who has had a heart attack to take an aspirin a day. However, a person with an aspirin allergy, a stomach ulcer, certain types of liver disease, or a high risk for bleeding should probably *not* take aspirin.

Unfortunately, the standard of care can be inadvertently overlooked. Some of my responsibilities have been to survey patient files to verify that all the patients were receiving quality care. I found that even the best doctor can miss something. We are all human and susceptible to making mistakes. For this reason, I recommend that you discuss all of the medicines or treatment options that are listed in this book with your doctor. Chances are that there is a good reason for why a treatment option is not being considered for you. There is no harm in mentioning this to your doctor and finding out why you are not a candidate for the treatment or medicine.

Chapter 5
Discovering You Have Heart Disease

There are three places where you can be when you find out that you have heart disease: in the doctor's office, en route to the hospital, or in the hospital. (Hopefully, only a few people have been told over the phone!) Occasionally, heart disease will be discovered during standard screening tests ordered by the doctor before symptoms ever develop. Usually, though, some heart-related symptom leads to several heart tests being performed (as described in chapter 3).

If a stress test is positive, that means that there is a high suspicion of heart disease. Angiography or a higher-level stress test will likely be recommended shortly after the results are known. Depending on the severity of the symptoms, there is usually no need for an immediate trip to the hospital. Your cardiologist will talk to you about what to do next. Many times the next step is to undergo an outpatient procedure within the next several days.

If someone has very severe chest pain, they may skip

seeing their doctor and go straight to the ER, where a battery of tests will be done more promptly. The standard tests will include an EKG, blood work, and vital signs. Blood work will measure levels of cardiac enzymes that are elevated during a heart attack. An EKG that shows significant changes and elevated cardiac enzymes means that the patient is having a heart attack or MI.

In some cases, the EKG is suspicious but the cardiac enzyme levels are only slightly above normal. This is called acute coronary syndrome (ACS), which is a general term for conditions that cause a lack of blood flow to the heart. In any suspicious case, a cardiologist will most likely be asked to evaluate the patient. Nearly everyone who is having a heart attack will require angiography to diagnose the cause of the heart attack. Only an interventional cardiologist can implant stents, but most cardiologists can diagnose heart disease and determine the extent of the disease.

Chapter 6
Dealing with the Discovery:
Stents, Bypass, or Medication?

No matter how you discover that you have heart disease, the question becomes "What do I do about it?" Remember that blockages are not considered significant until the arteries are 70 percent blocked or more (or 50 percent for the left main artery). You may have had CT angiography or invasive angiography that showed less than 70 percent stenosis in your heart arteries. In that case, your cardiologist may determine that no stents are needed, but you will be prescribed medication that will hopefully keep the plaque from getting worse.

If there are arteries blocked 70 percent or more, the treatment possibilities are balloon angioplasty, stent implantation, bypass surgery, or medication. Plain balloon angioplasty without placement of a stent is now rarely done. Angioplasty is the process of opening up the artery by inflating a tiny balloon at the site of the blockage. Essentially, the balloon just compresses the plaque against the sides of the artery but does not remove it.

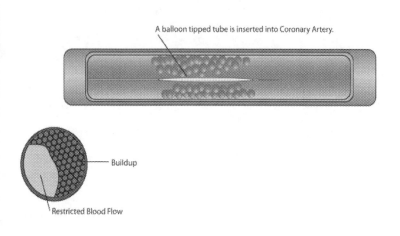

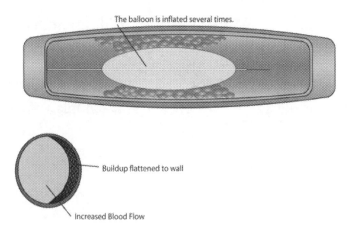

Angioplasty

After an artery has been opened with angioplasty, a stent is often implanted. Stents have been used since the early 1990s. A stent is a tiny tube of metal mesh that helps to keep the artery open. The two types of stents used are bare metal stent and drug-eluting stent. A bare metal stent is made up of metal only. A drug-eluting stent, or drug-coated stent, is a metal stent coated with a drug. The drug helps to keep the immune system from attacking the stent and allowing more plaque or another clot to build up at that site.

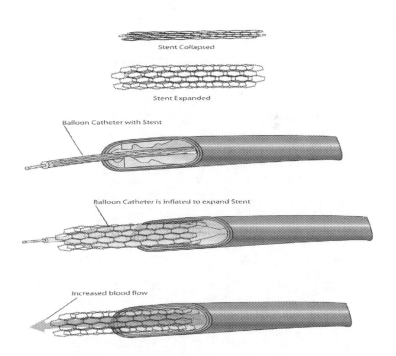

Stent

Sharon Masinelli, MCMS, PA-C

How does your doctor decide which type of stent to use?

Each patient is considered on an individual basis. This decision is rarely a black-and-white issue. Over the past decade or so, drug-eluting stents were preferred because studies showed that they had a lower chance of allowing a reblockage. The only major issue with drug-eluting stents is that a patient has to take an antiplatelet drug, such as Plavix (clopidogrel) or a brand-new drug called Effient (prasugrel). For this reason, bare metal stents were used for patients who had problems with bleeding, stomach ulcers, or other upcoming surgery.

In recent years, there has been some concern about the safety of drug-eluting stents. The medical community has debated whether to use drug-eluting stents at all since some cardiologists felt it might increase the risk of heart attack. However, a study published in 2009 found that there were no safety concerns with drug-eluting stents one year after implantation.[1]

Regardless of which stent is currently popular, your doctor is more likely to choose a bare metal stent if any of the following conditions exist:

- You will have major surgery soon and cannot take a "blood thinner" during the surgery

- You have a bleeding disorder
- You have a liver condition that causes problems with bleeding
- You are allergic to Plavix, Effient, or other antiplatelet medications
- You have a significant stomach ulcer
- You are not likely to take any medicines

How long does it take to recover after a stent implantation?

Recovery time varies based on the type of procedure and the extent of heart damage sustained. A person who had no problems during their hospitalization can go home after twenty-four hours and even return to work in one to two days. A person who experiences complications related to the stent procedure or who had a very large heart attack may need one to two weeks to recover. Many different factors are taken into account when estimating recovery time. Your doctor will tell you when you can leave the hospital, resume normal activities, and go back to work.

Sharon Masinelli, MCMS, PA-C

How does your doctor decide if you should undergo bypass surgery?

During angiography, a patient may be found to have extensive blockages. Severe disease may be defined as three or more blocked arteries. It may also be a blockage in a large main artery called the left main. Implanting a stent into this artery is a riskier procedure. Rather than attempting to place multiple stents or implant a stent in a risky location, your doctor may recommend coronary artery bypass grafting (CABG) surgery. CABG (pronounced as "cabbage") is a surgical procedure that requires cutting open the chest and sewing "new arteries" around the blocked arteries. Your cardiologist must refer you to a cardiothoracic surgeon for this surgery.

Bypass surgery is a much more serious undertaking than implanting a stent. The procedure starts as a minor surgery to extract "new arteries" from another area of the body (chest, arms, or legs) to transplant to the heart. Some of these "new arteries" are not actually arteries at all but veins from the legs or arms. Usually surgeons like to use the mammary artery in the chest.

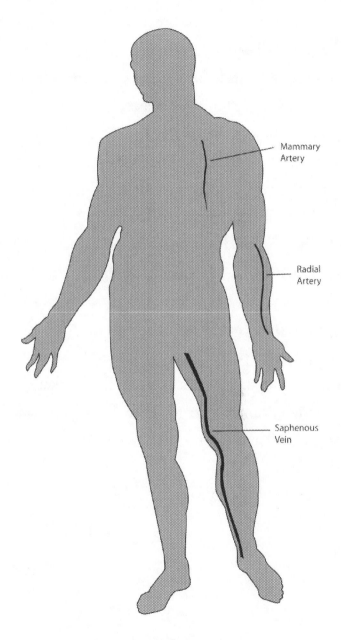

Mammary
Artery

Radial
Artery

Saphenous
Vein

Graft arteries taken

Sharon Masinelli, MCMS, PA-C

Once the "new arteries" are harvested, the major part of the surgery begins. Anesthesia is administered to all patients undergoing bypass surgery, and a breathing tube is inserted into the lungs. The chest is opened to expose the heart. Usually the surgeon must cut through the breastbone to get to the heart. Sometimes a minimally invasive approach is used when there is no need to cut through the middle of the chest. In either case, once the heart is exposed, the surgeon sews one end of the new artery onto the diseased artery just below a known blockage. The other end of the new artery is attached to the aorta, a large artery at the top of the heart. Hence, the blood flows from the top of the heart through the new artery and completely bypasses the blockage. After all the significant blockages have been bypassed, the chest is closed and stitched back together.

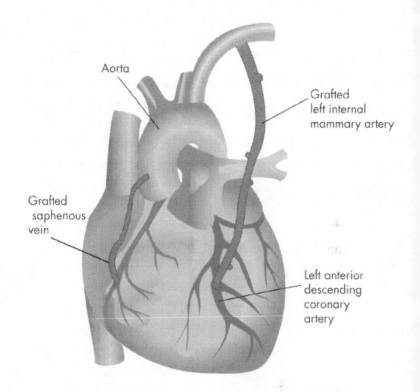

Bypassed arteries in the heart

Patients are often apprehensive and fearful of needing a bypass. Fortunately, better equipment and improved techniques produce better results, smaller scars, shorter surgery time, and quicker recovery. Minimally invasive and robotically assisted bypass surgeries are more widely available than ever. These types of surgeries can reduce the size of the scar to two inches and usually avoid cutting through the breastbone.

Many of my patients dreaded undergoing bypass surgery so much that they put off the surgery until the angina pain was unbearable. Usually within several months after the surgery, the patient would tell me that he or she wished the surgery had been done sooner. Certainly, the first few weeks were difficult, but overall, the experience was not nearly as terrible as had been expected. Plus, the results were excellent, and the patient could get back to doing normal activities without the fear of angina.

Chapter 7
What to Do after You Leave the Hospital

The most important thing you can do when you leave the hospital is to have your prescriptions filled as soon as possible. Do not wait one or two days before taking your prescribed medicines! Missing doses of certain medications can make things much worse for your heart (possibly leading to another heart attack or even death!). Everyone who leaves the hospital should be given a paper that lists their discharge instructions and medications. Verify that you are taking everything listed on your discharge sheet.

Look at the list of drug names on your discharge sheet and compare the names with the labels on the pill bottles the pharmacist gives you. If a medicine is missing, you may have been given a generic drug instead. The chart at the back of this book, "List of Common Heart Drugs," lists the brand and generic names for heart medicines. Use this chart to see if you have been given a generic drug. For example, your discharge sheet may list Toprol XL 200 mg daily. If you do not have a pill bottle that says Toprol, then look in the "List of Common Heart Drugs" table. You will see that metoprolol is the generic form of this drug. If you have a pill bottle marked metoprolol, then write this down on your discharge sheet so you know which medicine you have been given. Many times several of the dispensed drugs are generics instead of the exact medications listed on a patient's discharge sheet. If you find you are taking two of the same kind of medicine (such as both the brand and the generic), please call your cardiologist as soon as possible.

Once you have settled in at home, try to get more rest than usual during the first day. You should still get up several times throughout the day for short walks. Your body needs to recover, but you also need to keep the blood moving in your legs. People who lie down for long periods of time are at a higher risk of developing blood clots in their legs. These clots can travel to the lungs and cause a life-threatening problem called pulmonary embolus.

By your second or third day home, you should be feeling better and walking more every day. This is the time to prepare yourself for long-term care of your heart. You will need to follow through with a number of tasks.

1) Call your cardiologist's office and make a follow-up appointment. The discharge sheet will tell you when your doctor wants to see you in his or her office.

2) Create a list of every pill you take. This list needs to include medicines prescribed by your other doctors and all over-the-counter pills of any kind. People often forget to write down their vitamins or pain relievers, such as Motrin or Advil.

3) Evaluate your lifestyle and make changes. Most people know they should eat better, exercise more, and lose weight. Write down everything you eat so you can evaluate your diet. For the smokers, alcoholics and drug users, you know you absolutely must quit. No matter what your bad habit is, this is the best time to stop!

4) Buy a blood pressure monitor from the drugstore. A home monitor is very helpful for checking both blood pressure and heart rate. You should check the readings every so often as well as anytime you have a new health concern. Keeping your blood pressure and heart rate within normal range is vital to your heart care.

5) Sign up for cardiac rehab. Within the first several weeks that you are home, ask your cardiologist to

refer you to cardiac rehab. Cardiac rehabilitation is a special program for heart patients that lasts three to six months. You will exercise under the monitored care of cardiac nurses and trained staff. They will show you the types of activities that you should be doing and those that you should not be doing. Cardiac rehab is highly recommended for all patients with recent heart problems. Cardiac rehab is discussed further later in this book.

Chapter 8
Common Concerns during Recovery

After a Stent or Heart Attack

The most common complaints after a stent is implanted involve the puncture area for the angiography catheter. For most people, the catheter is introduced through a site in the upper thigh or groin area. The femoral artery is punctured with a large needle, and the catheter is guided up to the heart arteries. Because the femoral artery is a very large blood vessel, bleeding at the groin site is of some concern. Pressure is placed at the site after removal of the catheter sheath to stop any bleeding. A special closure device may also be used to help seal the hole and prevent significant bleeding. Closure devices can reduce the amount of time the patient has to lie flat after the catheter sheath is removed. Otherwise you may have to lie flat for four hours or longer.

Sharon Masinelli, MCMS, PA-C

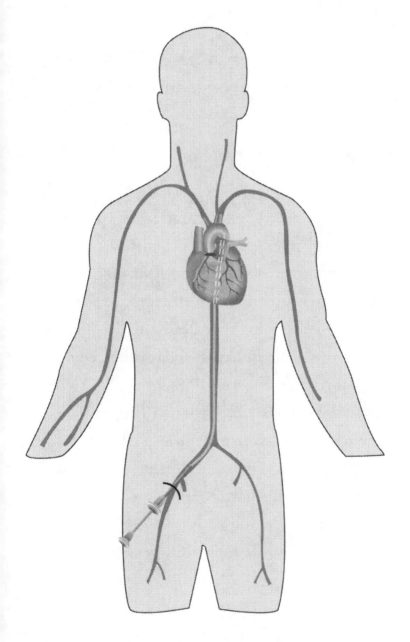

Groin puncture

Each hospital and doctor give different instructions and warning signs related to the stent procedure. Here is a list of some common instructions related to aftercare of the groin:

- A small walnut-sized lump at the wound can be normal if a special closure device was used.
- Do not soak in a tub for at least three to five days.
- Remove the bandage at home and gently clean the wound during a shower.
- Try to keep the wound dry after showering.
- Do not use lotions, powders, or over-the-counter ointments.
- No heavy lifting for three to five days.
- Some tenderness and mild bruising is normal.

Indications of a possible serious problem include the following:

- Fever
- Increasing tenderness, swelling, or redness at the wound
- Bleeding from the wound (soaking up a new bandage)
- Rash

- Severe chest pain
- Oozing of pus from the wound
- Throbbing mass at the wound
- Worsening pain, which may radiate to foot

Serious problems related to the stent procedure are rare. These include significant bleeding at the groin site, pseudoaneurysm, reblockage at the stent site, and infection. A pseudoaneurysm is when the tissue surrounding the femoral artery forms a wall and the blood flows outside of the artery. Surgery may be needed to fix the artery and prevent further bleeding.

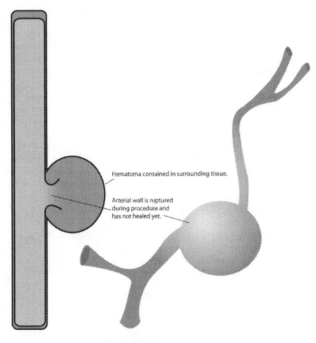

Hematoma contained in surrounding tissue.

Arterial wall is ruptured during procedure and has not healed yet.

Pseudoaneurysm

If you are concerned about a complication from the stent procedure, you should call your cardiologist. Many cardiology offices have an answering service that can address your concerns, even after office hours and on weekends. If you are very worried about a problem and cannot reach your doctor, you always have the option of going to the ER for evaluation and treatment. Most issues can be resolved with conservative treatments, such as antibiotics for infection.

Occasionally, patients will complain of feeling more chest pain after the stent is implanted. Do not be alarmed if you have very short episodes of chest pain. The type of chest pain of most concern will probably be similar to your heart attack or angina pain. If the new chest pain is different and lasts less than a few seconds, it is not likely to be related to blockages in the arteries. Always call your cardiologist if you are worried about your symptoms. If you experience severe, prolonged chest pain, call 911 immediately and take a nitroglycerin tablet.

Sharon Masinelli, MCMS, PA-C

After Bypass Surgery

As anyone can imagine, recovering from bypass surgery is a more involved process than recovering from a stent procedure. After the patient wakes up from the anesthesia, the breathing tube is removed. At various points during the first few days, the drainage tubes are also removed from the chest. Most people can expect to be in the hospital for at least four to five days while the chest wound is healing. Many complications are possible during the post-operative period. There are a number of complications that can slow down the recovery process:

- Abnormal heart rhythms, such as atrial fibrillation
- Infection of the wounds in the chest or artery harvest site
- Heart failure
- Kidney problems
- Low blood count or anemia
- Fluid surrounding the lungs
- Stroke

These types of complications can extend the hospital stay by one to two weeks or more. Most of the problems can be resolved simply with medication. Antibiotics are given for signs of infection. Antiarrhythmics are given for abnormal heart rhythms. Diuretics are given for heart failure or excess fluid surrounding the lungs. Patients with a very low blood count may need to receive one or more blood transfusions. Kidney problems may also require a change to the originally prescribed medications.

Once discharged home, you should be able to do some light activities. Patients are encouraged to get up for short walks daily to prevent deep venous thrombosis (DVT) or blood clots from forming in the legs. For patients who had conventional bypass surgery, most activity restrictions are recommended to allow the incision and breastbone to heal. Driving is prohibited for three to six weeks to prevent strain on the chest. Do not lift any objects that weigh more than five to ten pounds for approximately six weeks.

Pain at the incision site is normal. Strong pain medications (narcotics) are frequently prescribed for pain. The pain should be well controlled for the first one to two months. If you need to refill the prescription for pain medicine, call the cardiothoracic surgeon's office for a new prescription.

Some common discharge instructions related to bypass surgery include the following:

- Clean the incision gently during a shower.
- Do not use any lotions, powders, or over-the-counter ointments.
- Keep the incision site dry after showering.
- Avoid wearing clothes that rub tightly against the incision (bra, tight shirt, etc.).
- A slight clicking sound at the breastbone incision should go away completely in a few weeks.
- If you had the mammary artery removed, slight numbness or discomfort on that side of the chest is normal.
- A small bump at the top of the breastbone incision is normal.
- Take a laxative or stool softener as needed for constipation.
- Take a pain pill before bed to help you sleep better.

Serious problems for which you should call a doctor or go to the ER include the following:

- Fever

- Heart rate of 120 beats per minute or more when recorded by home blood pressure monitor
- Rapid weight gain
- Worsening shortness of breath
- Worsening pain, swelling, or redness at the incision
- Pus draining from an incision
- Rash
- Feeling as though you might faint
- Bleeding that saturates a new bandage
- Return of your previous chest pain or angina
- Sudden numbness or inability to move an area of your body

Many patients who have had recent bypass surgery experience poor appetite, trouble sleeping, and depression. These symptoms are normal and should improve over a few weeks. Undergoing bypass surgery is a major ordeal in a person's life. It makes you realize your mortality and the possibility of losing your current physical capabilities. People imagine that they will be severely disabled after the surgery. Considering that some people may not start to really feel better until nearly three months after the surgery, it's easy to imagine during that time that life will never be good again.

Sharon Masinelli, MCMS, PA-C

Recovering from major heart surgery can be depressing for just about anyone! Yet just when you think that you'll never feel better, your body starts to heal. You realize that you are able to do more and more activities without a problem. After three months of recovery, most people do not have significant complaints, and their quality of life has improved. In general, all regular activities may be resumed by three months after bypass surgery.

Swelling in the leg or arm from which a vein was taken is normal for an indefinite period of time. A lot of my patients would consistently get a little bit more swelling in their surgery leg compared to the other leg. Elevating the legs and wearing support hose help to reduce the swelling.

Regardless of complications and no matter how bad you feel, recovery from bypass surgery can be quicker and easier if you participate in cardiac rehab. The exercise and support patients get from cardiac rehab is proven to make them feel better.

Chapter 9
Staying Out of the Hospital

Whether you have had a heart attack, a stent implanted, bypass surgery, or just a heart scan that discovered significant heart disease, you should be on medication to reduce the chances of further plaque buildup! Too many patients seem to think that stents and surgery cure their heart disease. I cannot stress enough that there is no cure for heart disease. The term disease suggests a continuous process; in the setting of heart *disease*, this process is a continuous buildup of more plaque in the arteries. Bypass surgery and stent implantation can only help to relieve the worst blockages. Anyone with even minimal amounts of cardiology training can tell you that a person who has had heart disease symptoms in the past is highly likely to experience more symptoms in the future. Put simply, your body is prone to developing blockages in the arteries. Therefore, no matter what, any person who has had significant blockages needs to be on medication to prevent future problems. If you do not want to take a particular medicine, discuss this with your doctor to see if there is an alternative.

Why are medicines so important despite their potential problems? The reason is because the standard of care is to use certain drugs to treat heart disease. The standard of care was established by many experienced cardiologists and is based on strong scientific evidence. Evidence-based medicine is the backbone of any good cardiology practice. To be honest, you would be hard-pressed to find a cardiologist who does *not* recommend medication for heart disease.

You will find the same classes of drugs used for heart disease throughout the world. The World Health Organization (WHO) states on their Web site, "After a heart attack or stroke, the risk of a recurrence or death can be substantially lowered with a combination of drugs—statins to lower cholesterol, drugs to lower blood pressure, and aspirin."

The American Heart Association Web site states, "American College of Cardiology/American Heart Association guidelines recommend heart attack patients receive treatment with a beta-blocker, a statin cholesterol-lowering drug, an angiotensin-converting enzyme (ACE) inhibitor or angiotensin receptor blocker (ARB), and aspirin. A combination of the drugs has reduced coronary heart disease death by 80 percent compared to placebo."

Maybe you are still not convinced that taking medication is right for you. I can understand the hesitation to take pills that may have side effects. However, in my experience, people who understood the great benefits of the medicine were much more likely to tolerate them. At a cardiology conference in 2005, a large group of cardiologists was asked to raise their hand if they were personally taking a statin drug (Lipitor, Zocor, or Pravachol, to name a few). To my surprise, an overwhelming majority of the people in the room raised their hand! Essentially, cardiologists believe in these drugs so much that they take the drugs themselves to prevent heart disease.

Chapter 10
Types of Medicine

The type of medicine that will be prescribed for you is based on the scenario in which your heart disease was diagnosed. I will start with the basics that almost all heart disease patients are prescribed. I placed a heart in front of these medicines. After the basic medicines, I explain the drugs usually used in alternate situations and then the side effects of all the medications.

♥ Aspirin

Nearly everyone with heart disease should take an aspirin a day. The American Heart Association reports that a daily aspirin was shown to prevent another heart attack or stroke in almost 25 percent of patients. There are only a few cases in which aspirin is not beneficial. If you are *not* taking aspirin, you need to ask your doctor why. Aspirin is such a simple and important step that you can take to cut your risk by a quarter; however, not everyone can take aspirin safely.

Historically, aspirin is derived from the bark of a willow tree. The bark was used therapeutically for centuries before Bayer started selling aspirin in the chemical form in the late 1800s.

♥ Statin

These drugs are traditionally used to lower cholesterol. Crestor, Lipitor, Zocor, and Pravachol are different brands of statin drugs (more statins are listed in the "List of Common Heart Drugs" table at the back of this book). Many people believe that they do not need to take a statin because they have been told in the past by their family doctor that their cholesterol is fine. This is absolutely not true! Statins are given to people with heart disease regardless of cholesterol levels because they are proven to reduce the risk of recurrent heart attack and death. There are many large studies worldwide that support the use of statins in heart disease. For example, the LIPID trial (Long-term Intervention with Pravastatin in Ischaemic Disease), which began in 1989, studied more than nine thousand patients who were known to already have heart disease.[2] The study followed the patients for more than six years. The results showed that the risk of death from heart disease was reduced by 24 percent, the need for bypass surgery was reduced by 22 percent, the need for angioplasty was reduced by

19 percent, and the need for hospitalization related to angina was reduced by 12 percent.

Like aspirin, statins are also historically derived from nature. A naturally occurring statin is red yeast rice, or mevinolin. The substance used to make the first statin in the 1970s was produced by a mold called Aspergillus terreus. Researchers in Japan found that the mold's material could lower cholesterol levels in people. Statins work by decreasing the amount of cholesterol produced by your liver. We usually get plenty of cholesterol through our food, but your body also makes cholesterol. When the amount of cholesterol made in the liver is reduced, less cholesterol is in the blood.

♥ Beta-blocker

This important group of drugs used in the treatment of heart disease is traditionally used to treat high blood pressure. Toprol, Coreg, Tenormin, and Atenolol are a few beta-blockers (see the "List of Common Heart Drugs" table at the back of the book for more beta-blockers). The American College of Cardiology and the American Heart Association guidelines recommend that patients with known heart disease take a beta-blocker. One study published in the *New England Journal of*

Medicine in 1998 found that beta-blockers reduced the risk of death by 40 percent in patients who had had a recent heart attack.[3]

♥ Nitroglycerin

Patients with heart disease should always have nitroglycerin with them. It is an important medicine that can reduce or temporarily relieve the chest pain caused by heart disease. Nitroglycerin works by causing the veins to widen and lowers blood pressure. With a lower blood pressure, the heart does not have to work as hard to pump blood.

Nitroglycerin usually comes in a pill or spray. Patients are advised to carry the bottle with them everywhere, because when chest pain will occur cannot be predicted. For emergency relief of chest pain, you place one pill or spray one spritz of the drug under your tongue. If the pain is not relieved within five minutes, take another dose. If your pain is not relieved within another five minutes, then take a third dose, call 911 and chew an aspirin. Chest pain that is not relieved with three doses of nitroglycerin may be a heart attack.

Nitroglycerin is also available as a patch and as long-acting pills (Nitro-Dur, Nitro TD Patch, and Imdur).

These are used to treat chronic angina. Someone who continues to have regular chest pain despite treatment is often given a long-acting nitroglycerin to help minimize the pain.

ACE Inhibitor

These drugs are traditionally used to treat high blood pressure. ACE stands for angiotensin-converting enzyme. Altace, lisinopril, monopril, and Vasotec are ACE inhibitors (see the "List of Common Heart Drugs" table at the back for more ACE inhibitors). These drugs are more likely to be given to patients with heart failure as well as heart disease. The HOPE trial showed that high-risk patients taking the ACE inhibitor Altace had a 26 percent reduction in cardiovascular deaths. There were also 22 percent fewer heart attacks among these patients.[4]

Most importantly, patients with heart failure should be taking an ACE inhibitor. According to the CONSENSUS study, the chance of death was reduced by 40 percent after six months while taking an ACE inhibitor.[5]

Angiotensin Receptor Blocker

This medicine is a very similar drug to the ACE inhibitors. It works through a similar mechanism and may be used as a substitute when someone is unable to take an ACE inhibitor. Like ACE inhibitors, angiotensin receptor blockers (ARB for short) improve outcomes for patients with heart failure. A study called Val-HeFT showed that patients taking an ARB were significantly less likely to be hospitalized with heart failure.[6]

Antiplatelet

These drugs are commonly referred to as blood thinners. The most well-known brand name of antiplatelet medication is Plavix. A new drug called Effient is also now available as a substitute for Plavix. These medicines are actually like taking a super aspirin. They work by preventing platelets from sticking together to form a clot. As described previously, a heart attack is caused by the formation of a clot. Plavix or Effient help to reduce the chance of clots forming. According to a recent study called the CURE trial, Plavix decreased the chances of death, repeat heart attack, and stroke by 20 percent.[7]

If you had a drug-eluting stent placed in an artery

you should absolutely be taking an antiplatelet drug! Plavix or Effient is recommended for at least one year after receiving the stent. A missed dose can have serious consequences, such as an abrupt blockage in the stent and heart attack.

Stomach Acid Reducer

These drugs are traditionally used to treat heartburn or gastroesophageal reflux disease (GERD). One type of stomach acid reducer is a proton pump inhibitor (Prevacid, Prilosec, Protonix, and Nexium are some brands). A second, typically less expensive stomach acid reducer is an H2 blocker (Pepcid and Zantac are two brands of H2 blocker). Proton pump inhibitors and H2 blockers do not treat the heart directly but can be a very important drug in the treatment plan. First, they help to reduce the chance of bleeding from a stomach ulcer that can be caused by other medicines. Second, the drugs lower the risk of pain in the chest area caused by your stomach. Often the chest pain that causes patients to return to the hospital after a heart attack is heartburn or GERD, not another heart attack. If your doctor has prescribed a proton pump inhibitor, it is less likely that you will feel pain in your chest from the stomach.

Diuretic

These medicines are used most frequently for heart failure and swelling in the legs. Some commonly used diuretics are Lasix, furosemide, HCTZ (hydrochlorothiazide), spironolactone, and aldactone. Many people refer to these drugs as water pills. Diuretics help the body to get rid of excess water by stimulating frequent urination. One of the biggest problems for patients with heart failure is that fluid backs up into the lungs, belly, and legs. A diuretic can reduce the swelling and the shortness of breath caused by fluid buildup. These medicines are used to treat both short-term and long-term symptoms.

In some cases, a diuretic can increase your chance of survival. A study called RALES showed a 30 percent reduction in deaths for heart failure patients taking spironolactone daily.[8]

Digoxin

This drug was once commonly used to treat heart failure. Other names for the drug are Lanoxin and Digitek. Digoxin may work by slowing the heart rate and increasing contraction of the heart muscle. Doctors used to believe that digoxin would help heart failure patients live longer, but recently they discovered that this was not the case. However, it has been shown to help improve the quality of life for some patients. For this reason, digoxin is still beneficial for those with significant heart failure symptoms. It is also used to help slow the heart in the setting of atrial fibrillation.

Calcium Channel Blocker

This class of drugs has traditionally been used to treat high blood pressure. Examples of this type of medicine are Norvasc, Cardizem, and Procardia. Calcium channel blockers relax the blood vessels, which in turn lowers blood pressure. With a lower blood pressure, the heart does not need to work as hard. This is why calcium channel blockers are used to treat some cases of angina.

Side Effects

All medicines have some side effects. The list on a patient information sheet may seem endless. You certainly may break out in a rash from any medicine if you are allergic to it. Aside from that, here are some of the more common problems associated with taking heart medications that patients have reported to me.

- Aspirin may cause heartburn, upset stomach, and increased bleeding.
- Statins may cause muscle aches and increased liver enzymes.
- Beta-blockers may cause dizziness, fatigue, and slow heart rate.
- Nitroglycerin may cause headaches and dizziness.
- ACE inhibitors may cause a dry cough, increased potassium levels, and dizziness.
- Antiplatelet medicines may result in easy bruising and increased bleeding.
- Stomach acid reducers may cause nausea, gas, and diarrhea.
- Diuretics may cause dry mouth, thirstiness, headache, dizziness, and increased urination. Some diuretics may also cause decreased potassium levels, while others can increase potassium.
- Digoxin may cause nausea, diarrhea, and slow heart rate.
- Calcium channel blockers may cause constipation, swelling of the legs, and dizziness.

You should discuss significant side effects with your cardiologist. Do not stop taking a medicine without calling your doctor first! Everything you are taking is prescribed for a reason. Some medicines may need to be substituted if you cannot tolerate the side effects you are experiencing.

If you have questions about possible interactions of your particular medications, ask your pharmacist. If you need more information you can call the FDA (Food and Drug Administration) at 301-796-3400. The pharmaceutical companies generally have excellent descriptions of their medications on their Web sites as well.

Chapter 11
Vitamin Supplements Your Doctor May Like

Let's face it; there are a *ton* of supplements to choose from these days. Nutritional supplements claim to treat everything from fatigue to digestion to problems with urination. Yes, some are even designed to promote heart health. The question is how you know which ones are right for you. If you're not careful, you could be spending hundreds of dollars for unnecessary pills. I do not recommend taking very many supplements, because then people may forget to take their prescribed medicines. Nothing should replace your prescriptions! Instead, think of vitamins as a small thing you can do that *might* help in the fight against heart disease. In some cases they may make it a little easier for your medicines to do their job.

Keep in mind that the American Heart Association and many medical professionals do not officially recommend supplements. The opinion is that people should be eating a healthy diet that provides all the essential nutrients. Also, supplements are not regulated and may contain varying amounts of the active ingredient. If you are getting enough nutrients from your diet, there is no need for supplements. However, some supplements are considered better than others in the setting of heart disease. Supplements that are usually looked upon more favorably by cardiologists are niacin, red yeast rice, coenzyme Q10, vitamin D, fish oil, and omega-3 fatty acids.

Niacin is known to help raise your good cholesterol (see the next chapter for more information about niacin). Red yeast rice is the natural form of the cholesterol-lowering drugs known as statins and helps to lower your bad cholesterol levels. Coenzyme Q10 may help to reduce muscle cramps, a side effect of taking cholesterol lowering medications. Vitamin D deficiency increases the risk of heart disease therefore taking a vitamin D supplement helps to lower your future risk. Fish oil and omega-3 fatty acids help to lower your triglycerides and may help to reduce the risk of irregular heart rhythms.

Popular supplements that are *not* proven at this point to be helpful in heart disease are vitamin E, vitamin A, vitamin C, folic acid, and lycopene. Past studies may have suggested that these supplements are beneficial, but those conclusions have been highly disputed recently. Overall there is not enough evidence to support taking these supplements unless specifically recommended by your doctor.

Chapter 12
Cholesterol Basics

The way you look at your cholesterol numbers should change forever once you know that you have heart disease. A total cholesterol level of less than two hundred is no longer acceptable for patients with heart disease. In fact, your cardiologist will probably not pay much attention to the total cholesterol at all. The basic numbers they care about are LDL, HDL, and triglycerides.

One of the first steps in addressing long-term care of heart disease, from a cardiologist's point of view, is to lower LDL (low-density lipoprotein), known as the bad cholesterol. Your cardiologist will want the LDL to be one hundred or lower. Ideally, recent guidelines state that LDL should be less than seventy. If your LDL is too high, your doctor will probably consider increasing your cholesterol medicine.

After the LDL is one hundred (ideally, seventy) or lower, the focus may turn to HDL (high-density lipoprotein), known as the good cholesterol. HDL is measured at the same time as the other cholesterol levels. Your cardiologist will want to see the HDL levels as high as possible. According to the American Heart Association, an HDL level higher than sixty is considered protective against heart disease. In other words, you are less likely to have a heart attack or die of heart disease if your HDL is higher than sixty.

Current recommendations say to treat HDL to at least higher than forty. Unfortunately, there are very few drugs that help to increase HDL effectively. Niaspan is one of the better medicines and is a special formulation of vitamin B_3 called niacin. The most common side effect with niacin is flushing. Increasing the amount of exercise you do can also help to increase HDL.

The third important component of cholesterol levels is the triglycerides. Triglycerides go up when you eat a lot of carbohydrates and breads. Ideally, your cardiologist will try to get your triglycerides to 150 or less. Extremely high triglycerides may need to be treated first since, in some cases, high levels may inhibit accurate LDL readings. One of the most popular medicines for lowering triglycerides is Tricor. You should also try to reduce your intake of carbohydrates if your triglycerides are high. An example of a low-carbohydrate diet is the

Atkins diet. A recent study in Israel showed that low-carb diets can actually improve cholesterol profiles.[9]

During the treatment of high cholesterol, it is important to understand that the numbers will not improve overnight. Your doctor will need to wait at least one month before the effects of a cholesterol medicine can be seen accurately. Also, every time a change is made to your cholesterol pills, a new blood test will need to be taken within one to three months. Overall, correcting your cholesterol levels to perfection can be a lengthy process. Repeat testing will still need to be done at least every six months to a year even if your levels are perfect.

A small group of people have extremely high cholesterol caused by familial hypercholesterolemia. In these cases, the person has a genetic defect that does not allow LDL to leave the blood. Instead, the LDL continues to build up and is likely to be more than two hundred when measured in blood tests. Familial hypercholesterolemia can be difficult to treat, so adherence to your doctor's treatment plan is essential.

Chapter 13
Blood Pressure Control in Heart Disease

One of the most important things you can do to care for your heart is to keep your blood pressure under excellent control. High blood pressure makes your heart work harder to get the blood throughout the body. Most significantly, it increases your risk for a heart attack, stroke, and heart failure. A reasonable blood pressure is less than 140/90; ideally, less than 130/90. Newer guidelines set to be published in 2010 will likely suggest blood pressure should be maintained less than 120/80.

Many people have heard that an ideal pressure reading is 120/80, but you will find that your pressure varies on a daily basis. It is extremely rare for a person to have a blood pressure of exactly 120/80. If you can keep you blood pressure at 120/80, then you are doing an awesome job! However, if your pressure is frequently higher than 130/90, you should discuss increasing or changing some of your medicines with your cardiologist. The good news is that you are probably already taking a medication to lower your blood pressure. Most patients with heart disease are prescribed beta-blockers to lower their future risk of a heart attack. Beta-blockers lower blood pressure as well. This means that your doctor can increase your current medicine if you have problems with high blood pressure.

An easy way to check your blood pressure is by purchasing a home blood pressure monitor. They are available in most pharmacies and may be partially covered by insurance or Medicare if your doctor writes a prescription for one. Otherwise, they range in price from fifteen to one hundred dollars. The devices are easy to use and generally accurate. In order to make sure you are getting accurate readings, bring the blood pressure monitor in with you when you see your cardiologist. The office staff will check the readings and let you know if there is a problem.

Chapter 14
Cardiac Rehab

After a heart problem has been diagnosed, many people are anxious to return to their normal physical state. Some may bounce right back after a heart attack, whereas others feel that they may never do the same activities again. One of the best ways to improve your quality of life after a heart attack, stent implantation, or bypass surgery is to participate in cardiac rehabilitation (cardiac rehab). Cardiac rehab is a personalized treatment program that combines education, support, and exercise. Most patients view cardiac rehab as a three-to-six-month exercise program supervised by clinically trained staff.

Cardiac rehab begins with a referral from your cardiologist shortly after leaving the hospital. The rehab facility is typically on the hospital campus or near the cardiologist's office. At the first visit, a nurse or exercise physiologist will evaluate your capabilities and review your medical records. A class on nutrition and modifying your risk factors is usually included. You will often interact with other patients who have similar heart problems throughout your participation in the cardiac rehab program.

Once everything has been evaluated and discussed, an exercise routine is started. The exercise routine is done two to three times a week at the cardiac rehab facility. The rehab staff monitors each patient while exercising. Activities may include riding a stationary bicycle, walking on a treadmill, and lifting weights.

Chapter 15
Watching Out for the Signs of Heart Disease

Everyone with heart disease should know how to tell if they are having a problem with their heart. There are several key hints that can help you determine if something is wrong. Your heart may be in trouble if any of the following occur:

- You are experiencing pain that is the same or similar to your first heart problem
- You have discomfort or pain in your chest that worsens with exercise
- You feel a significant pressure or squeezing in the chest that lasts more than five minutes
- You have chest discomfort accompanied by sweating, nausea, and/or shortness of breath
- Your chest pain goes away after taking nitroglycerin
- You have significantly more shortness of breath with light activity

Remember, if you have crushing chest pain, you

should call 911 immediately! Any kind of chest pain is of concern. However, keep in mind that there are plenty of other problems that can cause chest pain. For instance, heartburn can sometimes mimic a heart attack. Try taking an antacid when you experience mild to moderate chest pain. If an antacid relieves your pain, it was probably related to heartburn. For more specific details on how to deal with chest pain, see the table "What to Do When You Have Chest Pain" at the back of this book.

One of the more common problems that can cause chest pain is something called chest wall pain. Chest wall pain is a harmless condition related to inflammation of the rib cartilage, chest muscles, or lining of the chest. If it hurts more to push down on any portion of your chest, you may be experiencing chest wall pain. Any movement of the arms that elicits pain in the chest is also probably related to a muscle problem, and not heart disease.

Chapter 16
Dealing with Heart Failure

Patients who have blockages in the arteries are more prone to developing heart failure. Sometimes heart failure means that the heart is not pumping enough blood to the rest of the body. This is called a cardiomyopathy (the word means heart muscle disease). The heart muscle is damaged by a heart attack, and the damaged muscle does not move properly, thereby weakening the heart.

A significant cardiomyopathy can be identified with a test called echocardiography. This test is a type of picture of the heart taken by transmitting sound waves through the chest. A cardiologist estimates your ejection fraction (EF) by looking at the picture, or echocardiogram. A normal EF means that 55–65 percent of the blood is being squeezed out of the left ventricle of the heart. If the EF is less than 50 percent, a cardiomyopathy is diagnosed and heart failure can occur.

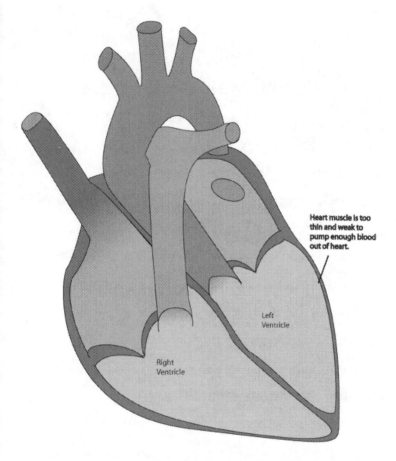

Heart muscle is too
thin and weak to
pump enough blood
out of heart.

Left
Ventricle

Right
Ventricle

Thin Heart Walls are a sign of systolic failure along with an EF of less than 50%.

Systolic failure

Sometimes heart failure can be a problem with muscle relaxation. When the heart does not relax properly, it cannot fill up with enough blood between heartbeats. In either case, blood is not moving forward well enough, and so fluid may back up into the belly, legs, and lungs.

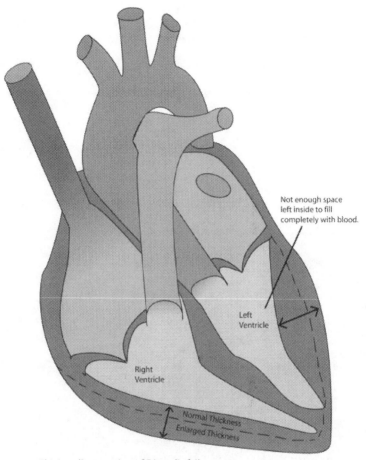

Not enough space left inside to fill completely with blood.

Left Ventricle

Right Ventricle

Normal Thickness

Enlarged Thickness

Thick walls are a sign of Diastolic failure.

Diastolic failure

Fluid in the belly causes your waist to swell and your appetite to decrease. Fluid in the legs causes the feet and shins to swell. Fluid in the lungs causes shortness of breath, which is much more noticeable when you are walking. The fluid in the lungs also makes it hard to breathe when lying down. You may feel as though you are suffocating at night while sleeping.

Many patients can live for years with heart failure. Modern technology and new medicines help patients live longer and have a better quality of life. If you have heart failure, being able to recognize what is happening is important so that you can keep the heart failure from getting worse. You should also know how to prevent future episodes of heart failure.

♥ What are the signs of heart failure?

Any of the following signs can indicate a heart failure problem.

- A weight gain of two to three pounds in one day or five pounds in one week
- Swelling in the feet and legs
- Swelling around the belly
- Worsening shortness of breath, especially when walking
- Inability to breathe easily when lying down
- Waking up during the night feeling short of breath
- Feeling very tired and confused

♥ How can I prevent my heart failure from getting worse?

Do not eat salt or anything with a lot of salt in it!

Read the nutrition facts label on everything you eat. Add up the amount of sodium (salt) that you eat each day. You should have no more than two thousand mg of sodium per day. Do not add salt to anything. You should also avoid eating fast food, pizza, TV dinners, and any canned foods. These items have a lot of salt and will likely make your heart failure worse. The safest foods to eat are fresh foods made without added salt.

Weigh yourself every day, and write it down on a chart.

Monitoring your weight carefully is one of the most important things that you can do to avoid going into the hospital because of heart failure. If you notice that your weight goes up by more than two pounds in one day or five pounds in one week, you should call your doctor. Increase your water pill (diuretic) if your doctor says it is okay.

Take your medications exactly the way your doctor has prescribed.

Several of the heart failure medicines are proven in studies to help you live longer. If you do not take them properly, you can make your heart failure worse. The dosages may need to be changed frequently in the beginning to find the dosage that is best for you. Once the medicines are at their proper dosages, they are more likely to strengthen your heart and keep you from going into the hospital because of worsening heart failure. A very important part of taking your medicines properly is ensuring that your cardiologist knows exactly what you are taking. Call your cardiologist if any changes are made to your medicines. Medicines may be changed to a cheaper form (such as a generic) at the pharmacy to save money. Your other doctors may also change the medicines you are taking for other health conditions.

Exercise several times a week.

People with heart failure *can* exercise. Try to set a regular routine for activity. If you have problems with joint pain, ask your cardiologist to refer you to physical therapy. A physical therapist can teach you how to strengthen your body for exercising.

See your cardiologist regularly.

Even if you are feeling well, you should continue to have regular checkups. There may be new or different treatment options available for you to discuss with your doctor such as a special pacemaker or other device.

♥ What could make my heart failure worse?

Illness or infection

People with heart failure will often have worse swelling and shortness of breath when they get a cold or infection.

Medicines

Several over-the-counter pills may make your heart failure symptoms worse. You should avoid taking anything like Aleve, naproxen, ibuprofen, Motrin, or Advil. Ask at your doctor's office before taking anything you buy at the store. There are also prescription medicines, such as corticosteroids and some diabetes medicines, that can cause problems when you have heart failure.

♥ When should I call the doctor?

You should call if you are feeling short of breath and your legs, feet, or belly are swelling. You should also call if you have gained more than two pounds in one day or five pounds in one week. Many people with heart failure take a medicine called a diuretic. You may need to increase the amount of diuretic you are taking to prevent worsening of your symptoms.

Chapter 17
Atrial Fibrillation

Atrial fibrillation (A-fib) is very common; it is an abnormal heart rhythm. A-fib is usually detected on an EKG. Your heart will suddenly beat quickly and erratically instead of beating at a regular pace. If you have A-fib, the electrical signals in the top chambers of the heart (the atria) are having problems by firing inconsistently. This causes the atria muscles to quiver rather than squeeze and pump blood. The bottom chambers (the ventricles) usually make up for the atria by still squeezing most of the blood out of the heart without a problem. Therefore, A-fib is not life threatening for most people. In fact, we are prone to developing A-fib as we get older. It is also frequently seen after undergoing bypass surgery.

The two most important problems that can be associated with A-fib are stroke and a fast heart rate. According to the Cleveland Clinic, a person with A-fib is five to seven times more likely to have a stroke. This is because the atria are not pumping properly. The blood that collects in the atria can form a clot that can break loose. If a clot breaks loose, it can travel to the brain and prevent blood from getting to an area of the brain. The best way to prevent a stroke related to A-fib is to take warfarin, a strong blood thinner better known by the name Coumadin. While taking this medicine, you will need to be monitored often by your doctor. A blood test should be done at least once a month to make sure you are taking the correct dosage. Unfortunately, many other drugs and foods affect how your body reacts to Coumadin. You will likely need to adjust the dosage several times.

The other main concern with A-fib is a fast heart rate. The ventricles may try to keep up with the atria, and they will beat quickly and erratically too. A fast heart rate for an extended period of time could cause heart failure. Most cardiologists prescribe medicines to help keep the heart rate below one hundred. Beta-blockers, digoxin, and calcium channel blockers are frequently used.

Chapter 18
Cardiac Diet

Dietary advice is difficult to give because the American diet is forever changing. There are so many options, and practically all of them are supported by a study. Initially, a low-fat diet was recommended for people with heart disease, because eating less fat meant lower cholesterol and lower risk of having a heart attack. Low-carbohydrate diets are currently largely popular with people trying to lose weight. A study released in 2008 showed that patients on low-carbohydrate and Mediterranean diets lost more weight and increased their good cholesterol more effectively than those on a low-fat diet.[9]

How do you pick a heart-healthy diet? With all of the diet propaganda, heart disease patients could easily be confused about what to eat. The first step is to start writing down everything you eat and drink. A study in 2008 by Kaiser Permanente showed that people who kept a food diary lost more weight.[10] Most people do not realize how much they are actually consuming until they see it in writing. Keeping a food diary also provides an incentive to avoid making poor food choices. You will probably feel guilty about indulging in that extra scoop of ice cream if you know that you have to write it down.

The next step to starting a heart-healthy diet is to show your food diary to your cardiologist. Have your cardiologist review your food diary and suggest improvements that you can make. If you feel strongly that you would like to start a particular type of diet, discuss the diet with your doctor at a follow-up visit. You will need to follow a diet plan that targets reduction of many of the following: calories, fat, sugar, sodium, and carbohydrates.

Also remember to look at the nutrition facts labels of your drinks. Most beverages contain enough calories, fat, sugar, sodium, and carbohydrates to ruin any good diet. Water is always the best option.

Five Healthy Eating Goals from the American Heart Association

1. **Eat more fruits and vegetables.** If you
   follow a 2000-calorie diet, aim to eat
   4–5 servings each of fruits and vegetables every

day. Vegetable or 100% fruit juice counts toward this goal.

2. **Eat more whole-grain foods.** Like fruits and vegetables, whole-grain foods are low in fat and cholesterol and high in fiber. Whole-grain foods include whole-wheat bread, rye bread, brown rice, and whole-grain cereal.

3. **Use olive, canola, corn, or safflower oil as your main cooking fat.** Limit how much fat or oil you use in cooking, and use liquid vegetable oils, such as these oils, in place of solid fats.

4. **Eat more chicken, fish, and beans than meat.** In general, skinless poultry, fish, and vegetable protein (such as beans) are lower in saturated fat and cholesterol than meat (beef, pork, and lamb).

5. **Read food labels to help you choose healthy foods.** Food labels provide information to help you make better food choices. Learn

what information to look for (such as sodium content) and how to find it quickly and easily.

Chapter 19
Quit Smoking

If you have heart disease *and* smoke cigarettes, your risk of dying from a heart attack is much greater. According to the American Heart Association, even nonsmokers who are exposed to second-hand tobacco smoke at home or work are up to 30 percent more likely to die from heart disease. The straight truth is this: smoking is bad for your heart! Smoking causes blood vessels to constrict and reduces blood flow to the heart. Smokers who quit lower their risk of heart disease by 50 percent after only one year.

Recovery from heart disease for smokers is much more difficult. Breaking the nicotine habit is almost never an easy task. Smoking is a very strong addiction that can consume a person's life. Quitting successfully can be easier with support from your doctor, friends, and family. You should start off by setting a quit date and letting everyone know about your plans to quit.

Your doctor can prescribe medicine to help you quit. Buproprion, sold as Zyban, is a medicine that has been prescribed for years to help some people stop smoking. One of the newest medications available is varenicline and is sold as Chantix. It works by blocking your body's nicotine receptors.

Smokefree.gov and www.chantix.com are Web sites that can help you quit smoking. Smokefree.gov is a government-sponsored free Web site. It offers a pamphlet you can print at home that will guide you through the process. Smokefree also has counselors available online and by telephone. The Chantix Web site is a twelve-week program that is available only to people using Chantix to quit smoking.

Chapter 20
Diabetes

If you have diabetes and heart disease, you need to keep your diabetes well controlled. Diabetes increases your risk of heart attack and stroke. You should keep your hemoglobin A1C below 7 percent in order to avoid increasing your risk even further. The hemoglobin A1C levels are usually measured as part of the blood tests ordered by a primary care physician for a regular checkup. These levels need to be checked every three months for the tightest possible control of diabetes.

Make sure you take your diabetes medications as instructed. Your primary care physician is generally responsible for prescribing your diabetes medications. A cardiologist specializes in treating only the heart and the cardiovascular system. Your cardiologist is not likely to write a prescription for diabetes medications or to order routine testing of your hemoglobin A1C level. You and your primary care physician have to make sure your diabetes is in check. If your diabetes is not well controlled, consider asking for a referral to an endocrinologist. Endocrinologists specialize in treating diabetes, hypothyroidism, and other hormonal disorders.

Chapter 21
Frequently Asked Questions

♥ When is it okay to have sex after a heart attack or heart surgery?

You should be able to resume having sex when you are able to resume your other normal physical activities. However, you should avoid sexual activity if you are feeling chest pain with exertion.

♥ Can I take Viagra?

You can take Viagra only if you are not taking nitrates at the same time. This includes nitroglycerin pills or any medicine with the word *nitrate* in its name. If you are not sure if you are taking a nitrate, you should ask your doctor or pharmacist. It is also very important that you check with your cardiologist before taking Viagra or a similar medication.

♥ What can I take as a pain reliever for headaches, backaches, or arthritis?

You can take acetaminophen, aspirin, or a short

trial of narcotics (the serious pain pills) as long as your cardiologist approves. Many recent trials have suggested that people with heart disease should avoid taking ibuprofen, diclofenac (Voltaren), and Celebrex. According to the American Heart Association, a medication like Celebrex could increase the risk of heart attack by 86 percent.

♥ I was told that I failed the six-minute walk test before I was released from the hospital. Now I have been given oxygen to use at home. How long will I need to use the oxygen, and how will I know if I can stop?

The most likely reason you need home oxygen is because your lungs are not working at full capacity yet. If you have a lung doctor (pulmonologist), schedule a follow-up with that doctor to discuss when you can stop using the oxygen. If you do not have a lung doctor, ask your cardiologist. No one can predict how long your lungs will need to recover.

♥ Will I need to take antibiotics when I go to the dentist?

Probably not. New guidelines recommend giving patients who have had a heart valve replaced or certain types of congenital heart disease antibiotics before dental procedures. People who have had a heart attack, a stent implanted, or bypass surgery generally do not need to take antibiotics before a dental procedure. However, you should ask your cardiologist to be sure.

♥ Will I need a stress test every year to check on my heart disease?

Guidelines currently do not recommend an annual stress test. For the most part, stress tests are done when you have symptoms that are of concern or you need clearance for surgery. However, some cardiologists prefer to have their patients undergo routine stress tests as part of a checkup.

♥ What do I do if my legs swell?

Elevate your legs, and try to limit the amount of salt in your diet. If you are also feeling increased shortness of breath, you should call your cardiologist's office for an early appointment.

♥ Can I take a calcium supplement with a calcium channel blocker?

Yes.

♥ Is it okay to take vitamins with my medicines?

Yes, but please review chapter 10, which discusses vitamin supplements. You should also tell your cardiologist about every vitamin that you take in case there is a potential interaction with your medicines.

♥ What should I do if I forget to take my medicines on time?

Take them as soon as you remember. If you are within a few hours of the next dose, then go ahead and wait until the next dosage time. Do not double up on your medicines unless specifically instructed by your cardiologist. Taking two of the same pills at the same time can cause significant problems.

♥ What do I do if I feel my heart racing (palpitations)?

Palpitations are very common and generally are benign. The first step is to sit down and check your pulse. Use your home blood pressure monitor to check your heart rate. Call your cardiologist or go to the ER if your heart rate is less than fifty or greater than one hundred. You should also seek medical attention if you get lightheaded, dizzy, sweaty, or nauseous with the palpitations. If your pulse is normal, with just a few skips here and there, there is no need to worry.

Chapter 22
Keep It Cheap

At some point during treatment for your heart disease, you may be faced with financial issues. Complaints about the high costs of prescription medications, heart tests, and doctor visits are commonly heard at cardiologists' offices. You probably now know that taking care of your heart can be costly! When someone mentions the high price of a medicine, I am reminded of what my grandmother said after paying for her cholesterol pills, "My doctor must think I'm rich!" On the contrary, doctors are well aware of how costly medicine and medical care can be and will usually try to help you keep costs as low as possible.

A constant struggle goes on behind the scenes at your cardiologist's office. Nurses and office staff spend hours a day dealing with pharmacies and insurance companies to make sure your tests and medicines are covered. A lot of this happens without the patient even knowing that there was ever a problem. Chances are that the staff at your cardiologist's office makes special efforts to help you get the care you need. For example, if you are suddenly unable to pay for a prescription, the office staff will often find samples for you and look into your qualifications for a prescription assistance program.

Frequently, your cardiologist can help you find a solution to your financial concerns. However, you usually have to be on your toes to make things work out perfectly. For example, you might find it is cheaper to get half of your medicines through a mail-order pharmacy and the other half from the local drug store. Here are a few ideas for getting your medicines at a lower cost.

Check out mail-order pharmacies for your prescriptions

The cost of many medicines may be significantly lower, the pills are dispensed in three-month supplies, and the prescriptions are delivered directly to you. Some examples of mail-order supply companies are Caremark and Express Scripts. Many local drugstores, such as Walgreens, will mail your prescriptions to your home as well. Research the costs of different companies by requesting price quotes or using an online service. If you decide to use a mail-order pharmacy, make sure your cardiologist gives you a prescription for a ninety-day supply!

Ask for generics

Many large retail stores, such as Wal-Mart, Target, Kroger, Walgreens, Sam's Club, Fred Meyers, Safeway, and BJ's, sell commonly used generic heart medicines for four dollars a month per prescription. Some will even sell you a three-month supply for only ten dollars. The biggest problem with this is getting the exact medicine that your cardiologist wants you to take. The generic form of some of your heart medicines may not be on the store's list (formulary). Make sure your doctor knows that you want to get your prescriptions from the four-dollar list. Keep in mind that you may find some of your medicines (like Plavix or Effient) are cheaper somewhere else if they are not on the four-dollar list.

Sign up for prescription assistance

Prescription assistance is when the pharmaceutical companies give you your medicines at low or no cost. This service is only available to people who cannot afford to pay for necessary medicines. Qualifications are based on your income. To find out if you qualify, go to a prescription assistance Web site or call your cardiologist's office. One of the more popular prescription assistance programs is Partnership for Prescription Assistance. The Web site is www.pparx.org, and the phone number is 1-888-4PPA-NOW.

Ask for samples of new medicines

Samples of more-expensive prescription medications are often available. You should ideally start a new medicine using samples and hold off from filling the prescription until you know that the medicine works well for you. After all, you don't want to find out after two days that you cannot tolerate the medicine or it is not effective for you after paying for a thirty-day supply. You would have paid for a lot of useless pills.

Enroll in a study

Cardiologists often participate in clinical trials and studies. These studies are frequently being conducted on new drugs for treating heart disease. If you qualify for a study, some of the doctor's visits, medicines, and tests may be free. Ask your cardiologist if you could be enrolled in a study for heart disease patients.

Chapter 23
Dealing with Insurance Companies

Occasionally, your cardiologist may want you to have a test or procedure that might not be covered by your health insurance. In these cases, you need to call your insurance company and find out if they will cover the test or procedure. For example, not all insurance plans will pay 100 percent of the bill for cardiac rehab. Your health plan may require you to pay a deductible and/or large co-pays if you decide to participate in the program. Many insurance companies will also refuse to pay for a coronary heart CT scan.

Your insurance company will be able to answer your questions more readily if you have the diagnosis codes and procedure codes. You will need to find out what the codes are from the cardiologist's office before proceeding. For instance, a diagnosis code for CAD (heart disease) is 414.00, and the procedure code for cardiac rehab is 93798. The codes have to be exactly as the insurance company requires or the company will not pay.

Here are facts your doctor's office wants you to know about your health insurance plan:

- Know what your insurance benefits are ahead of time. Specifically, is your cardiologist listed on your health insurance plan? Are they in-network or out-of-network? Does your insurance company require a referral from a primary physician?

- Whenever there is a question about coverage of a specific test or scan, call your health insurance company and ask if the test is covered. Document who you spoke with in case there are any problems later. To make sure the test is covered, you can request a precertification or authorization number.

Here are some lesser-known facts about Medicare:

- Medicare never pays for 100 percent of your health services! They pay 80 percent, and you get a bill from the doctor's office for the remaining balance.

- Medicare covers only a certain number of standard tests, such as pacemaker checks and cholesterol levels, per year. For example, you can have your cholesterol levels tested up to six times during the first year you are taking a statin drug. After the first year, Medicare pays for cholesterol checks three times per year. You will have to pay out of your own pocket for any additional cholesterol tests beyond this guideline limit.

- To find out if a test will be covered by Medicare, you can call 1-800-Medicare.

- Personal information regarding Medicare can be obtained by registering at www.medicare.gov.

Chapter 24
Finding the Right Cardiologist for You

One of the most important parts of your journey to a healthier heart is choosing a regular heart doctor. Heart doctors (cardiologists) can vary greatly. Even though most cardiologists follow the standard of care, each doctor's interpretation of the guidelines can lead to a wide range of treatment styles. Some cardiologists are more conservative. They prescribe a very minimal amount of medicines and schedule few follow-up visits. Others tend to be more aggressive in their treatment style; they prescribe more medicines and schedule frequent follow-up visits. You need to find a cardiologist with a management style that you are comfortable with. When it comes to your heart care, you do not have time to second-guess every move your doctor makes.

If you prefer a cardiologist who proactively adjusts his treatment plans to each update of the national guidelines and standard of care, I would recommend that you search several Web sites. First, go to www.ncqa. org, which is the Web site for the National Committee for Quality Assurance (NCQA). NCQA is a not-for-profit organization that promotes quality care for patients. You can search their database for the names of doctors who have passed the Heart/Stroke Recognition Program requirements. Look for the NCQA seal next to their names.

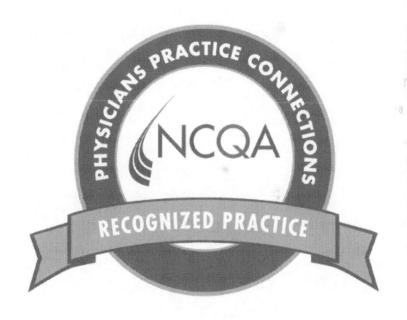

NCQA seal

Be aware that some of the doctors on this list are primary care physicians, not cardiologists. If you cannot find a cardiologist in your area in the NCQA database, then use an Internet search engine (Google, MSN, Yahoo, etc.) to look up cardiologists in your area. Use *cardiologist* and the name of the city you live in as key words. You can also use your local phone directory or ask a friend.

Once you have a list of possible cardiologists, check out their credentials. You can use the Internet, or you can call the American Board of Medical Specialties (1-866-ASK-ABMS) for information about a doctor's certification. On the Internet, you can review all types of information about any licensed provider through the state medical board's Web site. To find your state medical board's Web site, type in *State Medical Board* in any search engine and look for your particular state among the results. Physicians who have passed the cardiology board certification examination will generally have this in their listing under Specialty Board Certifications on the medical board's Web site. You might not want a doctor who is not board certified. The medical board's Web site can also tell you if doctors have had any lawsuits settled against them.

After checking out the doctors' credentials, the next step is to call the cardiologist's office for an appointment.

You will have to ask if they accept your insurance and if they are taking new patients. Many cardiologists practice in groups. If you really want to find the perfect match, consider asking the nurse, physician assistant, or nurse practitioner about the doctors. You might say, "I'm looking for a doctor who will see me often and treat my heart disease aggressively." Or you could say, "I'd like to see a doctor who is personable and open to alternative treatments." Chances are that they can guide you to the right doctor for you.

Chapter 25
Prognosis:
"Doc, am I going to live?"

You may feel as if having heart disease is like holding a ticking time bomb. Fortunately this can be far from the truth. In reality many people live long and healthy lives after discovering their heart problem. There are few cases in which a doctor will give a specific timeline or say that death is imminent within a few days, weeks, or months. This occurs most often to patients in the hospital. If you were released from the hospital, most likely your doctor feels that you are well on your way to recovery.

One of the more important factors when determining prognosis is how much damage was done to your heart. If there was significant damage, you may develop heart failure. Patients with severe symptoms of heart failure are more likely to have a shorter life expectancy. A recent study published by *JAMA* (*Journal of the American Medical Association*) found that people with heart failure were unaware of the seriousness of their prognosis[11]. Most patients felt that they would have an average lifespan and die at the national average age of death.

If you have an ejection fraction of 30 percent or less, you are considered to be at an increased risk of sudden death. Most people who die suddenly (without trauma) have an abnormal heart rhythm called ventricular fibrillation. Certainly this all sounds terrible, but there is some good news. In this situation, you can actually improve your prognosis! An implantable cardioverter defibrillator (ICD) can lower the risk of sudden death significantly and would certainly help improve your prognosis.

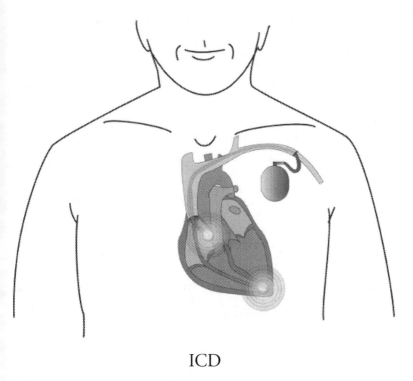

ICD

Anyone with heart disease should also encourage their friends and family members to learn how to perform cardiopulmonary resuscitation (CPR).

The question that most people think of is "When do I prepare for death?" The answer is always *now*! You can never know when things will take a turn for the worse. Prepare your living will while you have the ability to think properly. Do not wait until you are in the hospital again. Decide who should make medical decisions for you. Put your wishes in writing and make certain that that person understands your wishes. If you do not want to have CPR performed, then tell your doctor and the hospital staff as well.

Tables for Quick Reference

<u>**What to Do When You Have Chest Pain**</u>

♥ If the chest pain is very severe and crushing
- Call 911, place a nitroglycerin tablet under
- your tongue and chew an aspirin.

♥ If the chest pain is moderate
- Sit down and rest. Place a nitroglycerin tablet under your tongue.
  - If the pain subsides, call your cardiologist's office to inform them of your chest pain episode.
  - If the pain is not relieved within five minutes, place another nitroglycerin tablet under your tongue. If the pain is still not gone after another five minutes, take a third nitroglycerin tablet, call 911 and chew and aspirin.

♥ If the chest pain is very mild or barely noticeable
- Take an antacid, such as Tums or Maalox, to see if your discomfort improves.
- Make an appointment to discuss it with your cardiologist.

Basic Recommendations for Everyone with Heart Disease

- Take an aspirin a day.
- Take a statin drug every day (see drug list for examples).
- Take a beta-blocker every day (unless contraindicated).
- Take an ACE-inhibitor everyday if prescribed.
- Follow a specific schedule for taking your medicines (for example, take your medicines at 7:00 am and 7:00 pm every day).
- See your cardiologist frequently after leaving the hospital and then at least once every six to twelve months thereafter.
- Keep your LDL low (less than one hundred or seventy).
- Keep your HDL high (ideally, more than forty).
- Keep your blood pressure under excellent control (less than 140/90).
- Get involved in cardiac rehab.

- Exercise five days a week, for at least thirty minutes each time.
- Quit smoking.
- Eat a healthy diet.
- Keep your nitroglycerin close by.
- Limit your alcohol to 1-2 drinks per day.

<u>Five Important Things to Know about Your Heart</u>

1) **What is your ejection fraction?** Ejection fraction (EF) is the amount of blood pumped out of your heart. Echocardiography is most often used to determine EF, but angiography, cardiac MR (magnetic resonance) or a nuclear stress test can also be used to estimate EF. Normal EF is usually 55–65 percent. Anything less than 50 percent is considered low, and you may need to be monitored more closely. When the EF is 30 percent or less, your risk of sudden cardiac death is much higher. Frequently, medicines help to bring the EF up within three to six months. If it remains low, you should discuss with your doctor getting an implantable cardioverter defibrillator (ICD). An ICD will significantly decrease your risk of sudden death.

2) **Are your EKG results abnormal?** Plenty of patients with heart disease will have normal EKG results. Alternately, many patients without heart disease can have abnormal EKGs. You may be wondering why this is important. If someone with a history of heart disease goes to the ER because of chest pain, one of the first

tests that will be done is an EKG. If the results were normal before and have suddenly become abnormal, there is a higher likelihood that the person is having another heart problem. Doctors may be able to start treatment faster if you can tell them more about your usual EKG results. I highly recommend carrying a copy of your most recent EKG in your wallet so that doctors can have access to it quickly and easily.

3) **Have you had abnormal results on a stress test in the past?** This is important to know because it helps your doctor decide on the most appropriate test for your current situation. If you had a stress test that was abnormal before, then your doctor may want to proceed with a different test.

4) **What blockages do you have and where**? If you have undergone angiography or coronary CT, ask for a copy of the report and keep it with your records. A blockage of less than 70 percent is not considered to be significant unless it is found in the left main artery. However, a blockage or stenosis of 50 percent in any artery can easily progress to 70 percent or even 100

percent. Just because you did not need a stent last year, that does not mean that your arteries were clear. By knowing the extent of plaque buildup you have, you and your doctor can decide if and when more aggressive treatment is needed.

5) **Do you have a stent? If yes, how many and what type?** A lot of decisions regarding appropriate care are based on the type of stents that were implanted. There are two basic types: bare metal and drug-eluting. Drug-eluting stents have a chemical coating on the stent to help reduce the formation of scar tissue and clots at that site. Bare metal stents have no drug or chemical coating. With drug-eluting stents, it is very important that you take an antiplatelet medication, such as Plavix or Effient, every day for approximately one year, possibly for the rest of your life. Without the medication, you are at a higher risk of developing a clot in the artery with the stent that can result in a heart attack. So please make sure you know what type of stent you have!

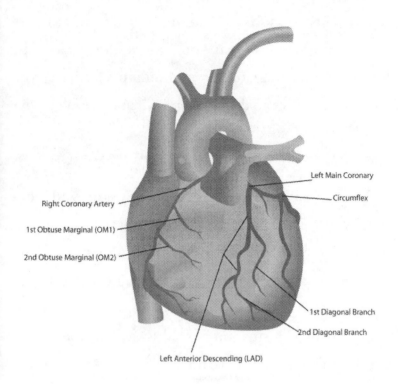

Left Main Coronary

Circumflex

Right Coronary Artery

1st Obtuse Marginal (OM1)

2nd Obtuse Marginal (OM2)

1st Diagonal Branch

2nd Diagonal Branch

Left Anterior Descending (LAD)

Arteries Found on the Front of the Heart

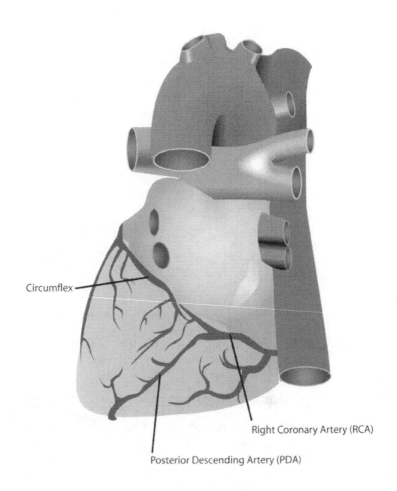

Circumflex

Right Coronary Artery (RCA)

Posterior Descending Artery (PDA)

Arteries Found on the Back of the Heart

<u>Interpreting Your Cardiac Catheterization Report</u>

- A blockage is called stenosis (or stenoses).
- Stenosis of 50 percent or more in the left main artery is severe.
- Stenosis of 70 percent or more in any other artery is severe.
- *Chronically occluded* means the blockage is severe but has likely been that way for a long time.
- Collaterals are when new arteries supply blood to an area that was previously not getting enough blood from a blocked artery.
- EF (ejection fraction) indicates how strong the heart is. Normal is between 55 percent and 65 percent.

<u>Helpful Tips for Follow-up Office Visits</u>

- Have your ID and health insurance card with you.
- Bring your pill bottles or a very accurate updated list of every pill you are taking, including vitamins and pain killers.
- Bring a list of your drug allergies.
- Bring a list of all your doctors (primary care, urologist, nephrologists, etc.). This will allow your cardiologist to send a copy of the office note to your other doctors. Sharing office notes is the only way all of your doctors can communicate with each other and work together to improve your health.
- Bring your weight chart and food diary with you, if you have one.
- Bring a list of questions you may have for the doctor.
- Do not put lotion or creams on your body the morning of your appointment.
- Verify with your doctor that you are taking all the appropriate medicines.

- Discuss your symptoms or concerns briefly with the nurse first and then in more detail with the doctor.
- Your doctor may make changes to your medicine. Write down the changes on your medicine list as soon as possible.
- Schedule your next follow-up appointment before you leave the doctor's office!

<u>What to Do if You Feel Lightheaded</u>

♥ Sit or lie down with your legs elevated.

♥ Take your blood pressure and heart rate with a home monitor. If your heart rate is less than fifty or greater than one hundred, call your cardiologist or go straight to the emergency room. Also go to the ER if your blood pressure is greater than 200/100.

♥ Separate your medicines if you are consistently lightheaded on a daily basis. Any medicines that lower blood pressure can be taken just before bed if needed. If they are causing your lightheadedness, the problem should be resolved once you take them at bedtime instead.

♥ Discuss your lightheadedness with your cardiologist. Some of your medicines may be changed to make you feel better.

♥ Have someone take you to the emergency room immediately if you pass out!

Items to Bring with You Wherever You Go

- Cardiologist's name and phone number
- List of drug allergies
- Medication list
- Nitroglycerin pills or spray
- Recent EKG

Weight Chart for Monitoring Heart Failure

<u>Date</u>	<u>Weight</u>	<u>Shortness of breath or swelling?</u>

<u>**Examples of Foods with High Salt Content**</u>

You should avoid or severely limit your consumption of these foods!

- Baked beans
- Baking soda
- Bouillon
- Chips
- Cold cut sandwich
- Cornmeal
- Fast food hamburger
- Fast food pancakes
- Fried shrimp
- Ham
- Hot dogs
- Macaroni and cheese
- Miso
- Pie crust
- Pizza
- Refried beans
- Seasoned bread crumbs
- Soup in a can (unless it states low-sodium)
- Spaghetti sauce in a jar or can

<u>Table of Vitamins and Supplements</u>*

Possibly more favorable to take if you have heart disease

- Coenzyme Q10
- Fish oil
- Niacin
- Omega-3 fatty acid
- Red yeast rice
- Vitamin D

Not currently proven to have a significant benefit

- Folic acid
- Lycopene
- Vitamin A
- Vitamin C
- Vitamin E

* Please remember that the American Heart Association does not recommend any supplements.

List of Common Heart Drugs

Brand name	Generic name	Drug Class	Action
Accupril	quinapril	ACE inhibitor	Lowers blood pressure
Accuretic	quinapril/hydrochlorothiazide	ACE inhibitor and diuretic	Lowers blood pressure and increases urination
Aceon	perindopril	ACE inhibitor	Lowers blood pressure
Aciphex	rabeprazole	Proton pump inhibitor	Decreases stomach acid
Adalat CC	nifedipine extended-release	Calcium channel blocker	Lowers blood pressure
Advicor	lovastatin/niacin	Statin and niacin	Lowers bad cholesterol and raises good cholesterol
Aldactazide	spironolactone/hydrochlorothiazide	Diuretic	Lowers blood pressure and increases urination

Brand name	Generic name	Drug Class	Action
Aldactone	spironolactone	Diuretic	Lowers blood pressure and increases urination
Altace	ramipril	ACE inhibitor	Lowers blood pressure
Apresoline	hydralazine	Vasodilator	Lowers blood pressure
Atacand	candesartan	Angiotensin receptor blocker	Lowers blood pressure
Avapro	irbesartan	Angiotensin receptor blocker	Lowers blood pressure
Axid	nizatidine	H2 blocker	Reduces stomach acid
Benicar	olmesartan	Angiotensin receptor blocker	Lowers blood pressure
Betapace	sotalol	Antiarrhythmic	Helps to keep the heart in normal rhythm
Bumex	bumetanide	Diuretic	Lowers blood pressure and increases urination

Brand name	Generic name	Drug Class	Action
Bystolic	nebivolol	Beta-blocker	Lowers blood pressure
Caduet	amlodipine/atorvastatin	Calcium channel blocker and statin	Lowers blood pressure and cholesterol
Calan	verapamil	Calcium channel blocker	Lowers blood pressure
Calan SR	verapamil extended-release	Calcium channel blocker	Lowers blood pressure
Capoten	captopril	ACE inhibitor	Lowers blood pressure
Capozide	captopril/hydrochlorothiazide	ACE inhibitor and diuretic	Lowers blood pressure
Cardizem	diltiazem	Calcium channel blocker	Lowers blood pressure
Cardizem CD	diltiazem extended-release	Calcium channel blocker	Lowers blood pressure
Cardura	doxazosin	Alpha-blocker	Lowers blood pressure

Brand name	Generic name	Drug Class	Action
Catapres	clonidine	Centrally acting alpha agonist	Lowers blood pressure
Colestid	colestipol	Bile acid sequestrant	Lowers cholesterol
Cordarone	amiodarone	Antiarrhythmic	Helps to keep the heart in normal rhythm
Coreg	carvedilol	Beta-blocker	Lowers blood pressure
Corgard	nadolol	Beta-blocker	Lowers blood pressure
Coumadin	warfarin	Anticoagulant	"Thins" the blood, prevents blood clots
Cozaar	losartan	Angiotensin receptor blocker	Lowers blood pressure
Crestor	rosuvastatin	Statin	Lowers cholesterol
Demadex	torsemide	Diuretic	Lowers blood pressure and increases urination

Brand name	Generic name	Drug Class	Action
Diovan	valsartan	Angiotensin receptor blocker	Lowers blood pressure
Dyazide	triamterene/hydrochlorothiazide	Diuretic	Lowers blood pressure and increases urination
Dynacirc	isradipine	Calcium channel blocker	Lowers blood pressure
Effient	prasugrel	Antiplatelet	Prevents clots in stent sites
Fosinopril	monopril	ACE inhibitor	Lowers blood pressure
Hytrin	terazosin	Alpha-blocker	Lowers blood pressure
Imdur	isosorbide mononitrate	Nitrate	Relieves chest pain caused by the heart
Inderal	propranolol	Beta-blocker	Lowers blood pressure
Inderal LA	propranolol extended-release	Beta-blocker	Lowers blood pressure

Brand name	Generic name	Drug Class	Action
Inspra	eplerenone	Diuretic	Lowers blood pressure and increases urination
Isordil	isosorbide dinitrate	Nitrate	Relieves chest pain caused by the heart
Jantoven	warfarin	Anticoagulant	"Thins" the blood, prevents blood clots
Lanoxin	digoxin	Cardiac glycoside	Slows heart rate, improves heart failure symptoms in some cases
Lasix	furosemide	Diuretic	Lowers blood pressure and increases urination
Lescol	fluvastatin	Statin	Lowers cholesterol
Lipitor	atorvastatin	Statin	Lowers cholesterol
Lofibra	fenofibrate	Fibrate	Lowers cholesterol
Lopid	gemfibrozil	Fibrate	Lowers cholesterol

Brand name	Generic name	Drug Class	Action
Lopressor	metoprolol	Beta-blocker	Lowers blood pressure
Lopressor HCT	metoprolol/ hydrochlorothiazide	Beta-blocker and diuretic	Lowers blood pressure and increases urination
Lotensin	benazepril	ACE inhibitor	Lowers blood pressure
Lotensin HCT	benazepril/ hydrochlorothiazide	ACE inhibitor and diuretic	Lowers blood pressure and increases urination
Lotrel	amlodipine/ benazepril	Calcium channel blocker and ACE inhibitor	Lowers blood pressure
Mavik	trandolapril	ACE inhibitor	Lowers blood pressure
Maxzide	triamterene/ hydrochlorothiazide	Diuretic	Lowers blood pressure and increases urination
Mevacor	lovastatin	Statin	Lowers cholesterol
Micardis	telmisartan	Angiotensin receptor blocker	Lowers blood pressure

Brand name	Generic name	Drug Class	Action
Microzide	hydrochlorothiazide	Diuretic	Lowers blood pressure and increases urination
Monopril	fosinopril	ACE inhibitor	Lowers blood pressure
Monopril-HCT	fosinopril/hydrochlorothiazide	ACE inhibitor and diuretic	Lowers blood pressure and increases urination
Nexium	esomeprazole	Proton pump inhibitor	Reduces stomach acid
Niaspan	niacin	Nicotinic acid	Raises good cholesterol
Nitrostat	nitroglycerin	Nitrate	Relieves chest pain caused by the heart
Norvasc	amlodipine	Calcium channel blocker	Lowers blood pressure
Pacerone	amiodarone	Antiarrhythmic	Helps to keep the heart in normal rhythm
Pepcid	famotidine	H2 blocker	Reduces stomach acid

Brand name	Generic name	Drug Class	Action
Plavix	clopidogrel	Antiplatelet	Prevents clots in stent sites
Plendil	felodipine extended-release	Calcium channel blocker	Lowers blood pressure
Pravachol	pravastatin	Statin	Lowers cholesterol
Prevacid	lansoprazole	Proton pump inhibitor	Reduces stomach acid
Prilosec	omeprazole	Proton pump inhibitor	Reduces stomach acid
Prinivil	lisinopril	ACE inhibitor	Lowers blood pressure
Procardia XL	nifedipine extended-release	Calcium channel blocker	Lowers blood pressure
Protonix	pantoprazole	Proton pump inhibitor	Reduces stomach acid
Questran	cholestyramine	Bile acid sequestrant	Lowers cholesterol

Brand name	Generic name	Drug Class	Action
Rythmol	propafenone	Antiarrhythmic	Helps to keep the heart in normal rhythm
Sular	nisoldipine	Calcium channel blocker	Lowers blood pressure
Tagamet	cimetidine	H2 blocker	Reduces stomach acid
Tambocor	flecainide	Antiarrhythmic	Helps to keep the heart in normal rhythm
Tekturna	aliskirin	Direct renin inhibitor	Lowers blood pressure
Tenoretic	atenolol/chlorthalidone	Beta-blocker and diuretic	Lowers blood pressure and increases urination
Tenormin	atenolol	Beta-blocker	Lowers blood pressure
Teveten	eprosartan	Angiotensin receptor blocker	Lowers blood pressure

Brand name	Generic name	Drug Class	Action
Teveten HCT	eprosartan-hydrochlorothiazide	Angiotensin receptor blocker and diuretic	Lowers blood pressure and increases urination
Tiazac	diltiazem extended-release	Calcium channel blocker	Lowers blood pressure
Tikosyn	dofetilide	Antiarrhythmic	Helps to keep the heart in normal rhythm
Toprol XL	metoprolol extended-release	Beta-blocker	Lowers blood pressure
Trandate	labetalol	Beta-blocker	Lowers blood pressure
Tricor	fenofibrate	Fibrate	Lowers cholesterol
Uniretic	moexipril/hydrochlorothiazide	ACE inhibitor and diuretic	Lowers blood pressure
Univasc	moexipril	ACE inhibitor	Lowers blood pressure

Brand name	Generic name	Drug Class	Action
Vaseretic	enalapril/hydrochlorothiazide	ACE inhibitor and diuretic	Lowers blood pressure
Vasotec	enalapril	ACE inhibitor	Lowers blood pressure
Verelan PM	verapamil extended-release	Calcium channel blocker	Lowers blood pressure
Vytorin	ezetimibe/simvastatin	Statin plus Zetia	Lowers cholesterol
Welchol	colesevelam	Bile acid sequestrant	Lowers cholesterol
Zantac	ranitidine	H2 blocker	Reduces stomach acid
Zaroxolyn	metolazone	Diuretic	Lowers blood pressure and increases urination
Zebeta	bisoprolol	Beta-blocker	Lowers blood pressure
Zegerid	omeprazole/sodium bicarbonate	Proton pump inhibitor	Reduces stomach acid

Brand name	Generic name	Drug Class	Action
Zestoretic	lisinopril/ hydrochlorothiazide	ACE inhibitor and diuretic	Lowers blood pressure and increases urination
Zestril	lisinopril	ACE inhibitor	Lowers blood pressure
Zetia	ezetimibe	Cholesterol absorption inhibitor	Lowers cholesterol
Ziac	bisoprolol/ hydrochlorothiazide	Beta-blocker and diuretic	Lowers blood pressure and increases urination
Zocor	simvastatin	Statin	Lowers cholesterol

Notes

1. Stone, GW, Lansky, AJ, Pocock, SJ, et al. Paclitaxel-eluting stents versus bare-metal stents in acute myocardial infarction. N Engl J Med 2009; 360:1946.

2. Prevention of cardiovascular events and death with pravastatin in patients with coronary heart disease and a broad range of initial cholesterol levels. The Long-Term Intervention with Pravastatin in Ischaemic Disease (LIPID) Study Group. N Engl J Med 1998; 339:1349.

3. Gottlieb, SS, McCarter, RJ, Vogel, RA. Effect of beta-blockade on mortality among high-risk and low-risk patients after myocardial infarction. N Engl J Med 1998; 339:489.

4. Yusuf, S, Sleight, P, Pogue, J, et al. Effects of an angiotensin-converting-enzyme inhibitor, ramipril, on cardiovascular events in high-risk patients. The Heart Outcomes Prevention Evaluation Study Investigators. N Engl J Med 2000; 342:145.

5. Effects of enalapril on mortality in severe congestive heart failure. Results of the Cooperative North Scandinavian Enalapril Survival Study (CONSENSUS). The CONSENSUS Trial Study Group. N Engl J Med 1987; 316:1429.

6. Maggioni, AP, Anand, I, Gottlieb, SO, et al. Effects of valsartan on morbidity and mortality in patients with heart failure not receiving angiotensin-converting enzyme inhibitors. J Am Coll Cardiol 2002; 40:1414.

7. Gerschutz, G, Bhatt, D. The CURE trial: using clopidogrel in acute coronary syndromes without ST-segment elevation. Cleve Clin J Med 2002; 69: 377.

8. Effectiveness of spironolactone added to an angiotensin-converting enzyme inhibitor and a loop diuretic for severe chronic congestive heart failure (the Randomized Aldactone Evaluation Study [RALES]). Am J Cardiol 1996; 78:902.

9. Shai I et al. for the Dietary Intervention Randomized Controlled Trial (DIRECT) Group. Weight loss with a low-carbohydrate, Mediterranean, or low-fat diet. N Engl J Med 2008 Jul 17; 359:229.

10. Hollis, J, Gullion,C, Stevens, V, et al. Weight Loss During the Intensive Intervention Phase of the Weight-Loss Maintenance Trial. Am J Prev Med 2008; 35:118.

11. Allen, L, Yager, J, Jonsson Funk, M, et al. Discordance Between Patient-Predicted and Model-Predicted Life Expectancy Among Ambulatory Patients With Heart Failure. JAMA, 2008; 299:2533.

Index